W0227830

Histological Typing of Tumours of the Eye and Its Adnexa

Springer
Berlin
Heidelberg
New York
Barcelona
Budapest
Hong Kong
London
Milan
Paris
Singapore
Tokyo

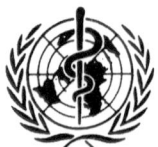 World Health Organization

The series *International Histological Classification of Tumours* consists of the following volumes. Each of these volumes – apart from volumes 1 and 2, which have already been revised – will appear in a revised edition within the next few years. Volumes of the current editions can be ordered through WHO, Distribution and Sales, Avenue Appia, CH-1211 Geneva 27.

1. Histological typing of lung tumours (1967, second edition 1981)
2. Histological typing of breast tumours (1968, second edition 1981)
9. Histological typing of ovarian tumours (1973)
10. Histological typing of urinary bladder tumours (1973)
14. Histological and cytological typing of neoplastic diseases of haematopoietic and lymphoid tissues (1976)
22. Histological typing of prostate tumours (1980)
23. Histological typing of endocrine tumours (1980)

A coded compendium of the International Histological Classification of Tumours (1978).

The following volumes have already appeared in a revised second edition with Springer-Verlag:
Histological Typing of Thyroid Tumours. Hedinger/Williams/Sobin (1988)
Histological Typing of Intestinal Tumours. Jass/Sobin (1989)
Histological Typing of Oesophageal and Gastric Tumours. Watanabe/Jass/Sobin (1990)
Histological Typing of Tumours of the Gallbladder and Extrahepatic Bile Ducts. Albores-Saavedra/Henson/Sobin (1990)
Histological Typing of Tumours of the Upper Respiratory Tract and Ear. Shanmugaratnam/Sobin (1981)
Histological Typing of Salivary Gland Tumours. Seifert (1991)
Histological Typing of Odontogenic Tumours. Kramer/Pindborg/Shear (1992)
Histological Typing of Tumours of the Central Nervous System. Kleihues/Burger/Scheithauer (1993)
Histological Typing of Bone Tumours. Schajowicz (1993)
Histological Typing of Soft Tissue Tumours. Weiss (1994)
Histological Typing of Female Genital Tract Tumours. Scully et al. (1994)
Histological Typing of Tumours of the Liver. Ishak et al. (1994)
Histological Typing of Tumours of the Exocrine Pancreas. Klöppel/Solcia/Longnecker/Capella/Sobin (1996)
Histological Typing of Skin Tumours. Heenan/Elder/Sobin (1996)
Histological Typing of Cancer and Precancer of the Oral Mucosa. Pindborg/Reichart/Smith/van der Waal (1997)
Histological Typing of Kidney Tumours. Mostofi/Davis (1998)
Histological Typing of Testis Tumours. Mostofi/Sesterhenn (1998)
Histological Typing of Tumours of the Eye and Its Adnexa. Campbell (1998)

Histological Typing
of Tumours
of the Eye and Its Adnexa

R.J. Campbell

In Collaboration with L.H. Sobin
and Pathologists in 11 Countries

Second Edition

With 112 Colour Figures

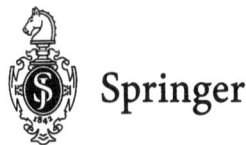 Springer

Jean Campbell, MD
Professor of Pathology
Departments of Ophthalmology and Pathology
Mayo Clinic, 200 First Street, SW
Rochester, MN 55905, USA

L.H. Sobin, MD
Head, WHO Collaborating Center for the
International Histological Classification of Tumours
Armed Forces Institute of Pathology
Washington, DC 20306-6000, USA

First edition published by WHO in 1980 as No. 24 in the International Histological Classification of Tumours series

ISBN-13:978-3-540-64131-5

Library of Congress Cataloging-in-Publication Data
Campbell, R.J. (R. Jean), 1934 – Histological typing of tumours of the eye and its adnexa / R.J.
Campbell; in collaboration with pathologists in 11 countries. – 2nd ed. p. cm. – (International histo-
logical classification of tumours)
Rev. ed. of: Histological typing of tumours of the eye and its adnexa / L.E. Zimmermann, in collabo-
ration with L.H. Sobin and pathologists in 13 countries. 1980. Includes bibliographical references and
index.
ISBN-13:978-3-540-64131-5   e-ISBN-13:978-3-642-72163-2
DOI: 10.1007/978-3-642-72163-2

1. Eye -Tumours -Histopathology -Atlases. 2. Eye-Tumours-Classification. 3. Adnexa oculi-Tumours-
Classification. I. Zimmermann, L.E. (Lorenz E.) Histological typing of tumours of the eye and its
adnexa. II. Series: International histological classification of tumours (Unnumbered) [DNLM: 1. Eye
Neoplasms-pathology. 2. Eye Neoplasms-classification. WW 149C189h 1998]   RC280.E9C36
1998 616.99'28407583–dc21 DNLM/DLC   98-26176

This work is subject to copyright. All rights are reserved, whether the whole or part of the material is
concerned, specifically the rights of translation, reprinting, reuse of illustrations, recitation, broad-
casting, reproduction on microfilm or in any other ways, and storage in data banks. Duplication of this
publication or parts thereof is permitted only under the provisions of the German Copyright Law of
September 9, 1965, in its current version, and permission for use must always be obtained from
Springer-Verlag. Violations are liable for prosecution under the German Copyright Law.

© Springer-Verlag Berlin Heidelberg 1998

The use of general descriptive names, registered names, trademarks, etc. in this publication does not
imply, even in the absence of a specific statement, that such names are exempt from the relevant pro-
tective laws and regulations and therefore free for general use.

Product liability: The publisher cannot guarantee the accuracy of any information about dosage and
application contained in this book. In every individual case the user must check such information by
consulting the relevant literature.

Typesetting: Springer-Verlag, Heidelberg, Margot Weichhold

SPIN: 10667058   81/3135 – 5 4 3 2 1 0 – Printed on acid-free paper

Participants

Burnier, Miguel N. Jr., Dr.
Departments of Ophthalmology and Pathology,
Royal Victoria Hospital, Montreal, Quebec, Canada

Campbell, R. Jean, Dr.
Departments of Ophthalmology and Pathology,
Mayo Clinic, Rochester, Minnesota, USA

Croxatto, J. Oscar, Dr.
Department of Pathology, Fundacion Oftalmologica,
Jorge Malbran, Buenos Aires, Argentina

Lee, William R., Dr.
Department of Pathology, University of Glasgow,
Western Infirmary, Glasgow, Scotland

McLean, Ian W., Dr.
Department of Ophthalmic Pathology, Armed Forces Institute
of Pathology, Washington, DC, USA

Naumann, G.O.H., Dr.
Friedrich-Alexander-Universität, Erlangen-Nürnberg,
Augenklinik mit Poliklinik, Erlangen, Germany

Pe'er, Jacob, Dr.
Hadassah University Hospital, Hebrew-University Hadassah
Medical School, Jerusalem, Israel

Prause, J.U., Dr.
Eye Pathology Institute, University of Copenhagen, Denmark

Sahel, José, Dr.
Université Louis Pasteur, Strasbourg, France

Sobin, Leslie H., Dr.
Armed Forces Institute of Pathology, Washington, DC, USA

Tarkkanen, Ahti, Dr.
Department of Ophthalmology, University of Helsinki,
Helsinki, Finland

Tso, Mark O.M., Dr.
Departments of Ophthalmology and Visual Sciences,
The Chinese University of Hong Kong, Prince of Wales Hospital,
Shatin, New Territories, Hong Kong

Uyama, Masanobu, Dr.
Department of Ophthalmology, Kansai Medical University,
Osaka, Japan

General Preface to the Series

Among the prerequisites for comparative studies of cancer are international agreement on histological criteria for the definition and classification of cancer types and a standardized nomenclature. An internationally agreed classification of tumours, acceptable to physicians, surgeons, radiologists, pathologists and statisticians alike, would enable cancer workers in all parts of the world to compare their findings and would facilitate collaboration among them.

In a report published in 1952[1], a subcommittee of the World Health Organization (WHO) Expert Committee on Health Statistics discussed the general principles that should govern the statistical classification of tumours and agreed that, to ensure the necessary flexibility and ease of coding, three separate classifications were needed according to (1) anatomical site, (2) histological type and (3) degree of malignancy. A classification according to anatomical site is available in the International Classification of Diseases[2].

In 1956, the WHO Executive Board passed a resolution[3] requesting the Director-General to explore the possibility that WHO might organize centres in various parts of the world and arrange for the collection of human tissues and their histological classification. The main purpose of such centres would be to develop histological definitions of cancer types and to facilitate the wide adoption of a uniform nomenclature. The resolution was endorsed by the Tenth World Health Assembly in May 1957[4].

---

[1] WHO (1952) WHO Technical Report Series. No. 53, 1952, p. 45
[2] WHO (1977) Manual of the international statistical classification of diseases, injuries, and causes of death. 1975 version. WHO, Geneva
[3] WHO (1956) WHO Official Records. No. 68, p. 14 (resolution EB 17.R40)
[4] WHO (1957) WHO Official Records. No. 79, p. 467 (resolution WHA 10.18)

Since 1958, WHO has established a number of centres concerned with this subject. The result of this endeavour has been
the International Histological Classification of Tumours, a multi-
volume series whose first edition was published between 1967
and 1981. The present revised second edition aims to update the
classification, reflecting progress in diagnosis and the relevance
of tumour types to clinical and epidemiological features.

Preface to Histological Typing of Tumours of the Eye and Its Adnexa, Second Edition

The first edition of *Histological Typing of Tumours of the Eye and Its Adnexa*[1] was the result of a collaborative effort organized by WHO in 1972. Pathologists from eight countries participated in this effort, and an additional six pathologists from other countries reviewed the material. The classification was published in 1980.

In order to update the classification, a panel was formed with new and former members of the WHO group. Technological advances in pathology have been incorporated and reflect the current state of our knowledge. Modifications will be needed as experience accumulates. Although the present classification has been adopted by the members of the group, it necessarily represents a view from which some pathologists may wish to dissent. It is hoped that, in the interests of international cooperation, all pathologists would use the classification that is presented. Criticisms and suggestions for its improvement will be welcomed; these should be sent to the World Health Organization, 1211 Geneva 27, Switzerland.

The publications in the series *International Histological Classification of Tumours* are not intended to serve as textbooks, but rather to promote the adoption of a uniform terminology that will facilitate communication among cancer workers. For this reason, the literature references have been intentionally omitted and readers should refer to standard works for bibliographies.

---

[1] Zimmerman LE (1980) Histological typing of tumours of the eye and its adnexa. World Health Organization, Geneva

Contents

Introduction

Since the first edition of *Histological Typing of Tumours of the Eye and Its Adnexa*, published in 1980, immunohistochemistry and findings in molecular biology have contributed to our knowledge of the histogenesis of many tumours. These findings have been incorporated in this current text. The classification has been confined largely to true neoplasms. Tumour-like lesions (e.g. reactive lymphoid hyperplasia, pterygium, telangiectasia) are grouped with the benign tumours. Changes in nomenclature reflect an update in knowledge of morphological identification of cell types, behavioural patterns and clinico-pathological correlations.

Definitions are given for lesions specific to the eye and its adnexa. For other lesions, the definitions of the relevant WHO classifications for the skin, soft tissues, salivary glands and nervous system should be used. Until the revised WHO lymphoma classification is available, the NCI working formulation, the updated Kiel classification or the REAL classification are recommended.

Histological Classification of Tumours of the Eye and Its Adnexa

Tumours of the Eyelid

The tumours that are listed include those that are commonly found in the eye as well as rarer entities that have been described in the past decade. In all instances, the reader is referred to the WHO Histological Typing of Skin Tumours.

1 Epithelial Tumours

1.1 Benign
1.1.1   Squamous cell papilloma
1.1.2   Seborrhoeic keratosis
1.1.3   Inverted follicular keratosis
1.1.4   Keratoacanthoma
1.1.5   Reactive hyperplasia (pseudoepitheliomatous hyperplasia)
1.1.6   Sebaceous gland hyperplasia
1.1.7   Sebaceous gland adenoma
1.1.8   Trichoepithelioma
1.1.9   Trichofolliculoma
1.1.10 Trichilemmoma
1.1.11 Pilomatrixoma
1.1.12 Other tumours of hair follicles
1.1.13 Syringoma
1.1.14 Papillary syringadenoma
1.1.15 Eccrine spiradenoma
1.1.16 Eccrine acrospiroma
1.1.17 Pleomorphic adenoma
1.1.18 Eccrine cylindroma
1.1.19 Hydrocystoma

1.1.20 Apocrine adenoma
1.1.21 Other benign sweat gland tumours
1.1.22 Retention cyst
1.1.23 Trichilemmal cyst
1.1.24 Epidermal cyst
1.1.25 Other benign cystic lesions
1.1.26 Junctional naevus
1.1.27 Intradermal naevus
1.1.28 Compound naevus
1.1.29 Spitz naevus (epithelioid and/or spindle cell naevus)
1.1.30 Balloon cell naevus
1.1.31 Blue naevus
1.1.32 Cellular blue naevus
1.1.33 Naevus of Ota
1.1.34 Congenital dysplastic naevus
1.1.35 Xanthelasma

1.2   *Precancerous*
1.2.1   Actinic keratosis
1.2.2   Intraepithelial neoplasia (Bowen disease)
1.2.3   Radiation dermatosis
1.2.4   Xeroderma pigmentosum

1.3   *Malignant*
1.3.1   Squamous cell carcinoma
1.3.2   Basal cell carcinoma

1.3.3   Sebaceous gland carcinoma (Figs. 1–4)
A malignant tumour with some degree of sebaceous differentiation.
    Atypical cells show cytoplasmic vacuolization to a variable degree and have a vesicular nucleus.
    An anaplastic form with minimally vacuolated cells may be confused with squamous cell carcinoma or basal cell carcinoma. Intracytoplasmic fat can be demonstrated on frozen tissue with the oil red-O stain. Cells are arranged in groups or nodules that may show a central area of necrosis. Highly infiltrating tumours may grow as broad sheets of cells.
    Tumour cells may be present in the surface epithelium as Paget cells. Intraepithelial spread can simulate in situ carcinoma.
    Sebaceous gland carcinoma is more common in the eyelid than in any other part of the skin. It arises from the meibomian glands or the glands of Zeis. The tumour is more common in the upper lid, where these glands are most numerous.

1.3.4   Carcinoma of hair follicles
1.3.5   Sweat gland adenocarcinoma

1.3.6   Merkel cell tumour (Figs. 5, 6)
A relatively rare malignant neoplasm that arises from precursor cells of keratinocytes and Merkel cells.

Cells with round to oval nuclei, inconspicuous nucleoli and scanty cytoplasm are arranged in diffuse sheets or a trabecular pattern. Pseudorosettes or a pseudoglandular pattern occurs. Mitotic figures are usually numerous. The diagnostically useful antigenic profiles include simple epithelial cytokeratins 8, 18 and 20 in addition to neurofilament triplet proteins, chromogranin and synaptophysin. Met-enkephalin and other neuropeptides are present in a subset of these tumours. The salient findings on transmission electron microscopy are the presence of dense-core neurosecretory granules and perinuclear whorls of intermediate filaments.

This tumour has a predilection for the upper eyelid of elderly women and may grow rapidly with spread to regional lymph nodes.

1.3.7   Melanoma arising from naevi
1.3.8   Melanoma arising in primary acquired melanosis
            with atypia
1.3.9   Melanoma arising de novo

2   **Fibrous Tissue Tumours**

2.1   Benign
2.1.1   Fibroma
2.1.2   Keloid
2.1.3   Nodular fasciitis
2.1.4   Proliferative fasciitis
2.1.5   Others

2.2   Fibromatosis
2.2.1   Superficial
2.2.2   Deep

2.3   Malignant
2.3.1   Fibrosarcoma
2.3.2   Congenital fibrosarcoma
2.3.3   Others, e.g. malignant fibrous tumour

3   Fibrohistiocytic Tumours

3.1   Benign
3.1.1   Dermatofibroma
3.1.2   Juvenile xanthogranuloma
3.1.3   Reticulohistiocytoma
3.1.4   Xanthoma

3.2   Intermediate
3.2.1   Atypical fibroxanthoma
3.2.2   Dermatofibrosarcoma protruberans
3.2.3   Others, e.g. angiomatoid fibrous histiocytoma

3.3   Malignant
3.3.1   Malignant fibrous histiocytoma
3.3.2   Malignant fibroxanthoma
3.3.3   Others, e.g. malignant giant cell fibrous histiocytoma

4   Lipomatous Tumours

4.1   Benign
4.1.1   Lipoma
4.1.2   Others, e.g. hibernoma

4.2   Malignant
4.2.1   Liposarcoma

5   Smooth Muscle Tumours

5.1   Benign
5.1.1   Leiomyoma
5.1.2   Angiomyoma

5.2   Malignant
5.2.1   Leiomyosarcoma

6   Skeletal Muscle Tumours

6.1   Benign
6.1.1   Rhabdomyoma

6.2   Malignant
6.2.1   Rhabdomyosarcoma, embryonal
6.2.2   Rhabdomyosarcoma, spindle cell
6.2.3   Rhabdomyosarcoma, alveolar
6.2.4   Rhabdomyosarcoma, pleomorphic

7   Endothelial Tumours

7.1   Benign
7.1.1   Papillary endothelial hyperplasia
7.1.2   Capillary haemangioma
7.1.3   Cavernous haemangioma
7.1.4   Venous haemangioma
7.1.5   Epithelioid haemangioma (angiolymphoid hyperplasia)
7.1.6   Pyogenic granuloma (exuberant granulation type)
7.1.7   Lymphangioma
7.1.8   Others

7.2   Malignant
7.2.1   Angiosarcoma
7.2.2   Lymphangiosarcoma
7.2.3   Kaposi sarcoma

8   Perivascular Tumours

8.1   Benign
8.1.1   Haemangiopericytoma
8.1.2   Glomus tumour

8.2   Malignant
8.2.1   Malignant haemangiopericytoma
8.2.2   Malignant glomus tumour

9   Neural Tumours

9.1   Benign
9.1.1   Neurofibroma
9.1.2   Traumatic neuroma
9.1.3   Plexiform neurofibroma
9.1.4   Schwannoma
9.1.5   Others, e.g. neuroglial choristoma
        (heterotopic neuroglial tissue)

9.2   Malignant
9.2.1   Malignant peripheral nerve sheath tumour (MPNST)

10   Cartilage and Bone Tumours

10.1   Benign
10.1.1 Chondroma
10.1.2 Osteoma

10.2   Malignant
10.2.1 Chondrosarcoma
10.2.2 Mesenchymal chondrosarcoma
10.2.3 Osteosarcoma

11   Hamartomas, Choristomas and Miscellaneous Tumours

11.1.1 Dermoid cyst
A dermoid cyst may present in the eyelid but more typically occurs as an orbital mass.

11.1.2 Phakomatous choristoma (Zimmerman tumour)
        (Figs. 7–10)
A lenticular anlage in the subcutaneous tissue and dermis of the lower nasal eyelid.

Thick basement membrane surrounds small nests of cuboidal cells that lie in a dense collagenous matrix. Some cells resemble "bladder" cells. Excrescences of basement membrane often project into the epithelial islands. Foci of dystrophic calcification and psammoma-like bodies may be present. The entity is rare and appears as an enlarging nodule within the first 6 months of life.

11.1.3 Myxoma (Fig. 11)
This is a non-encapsulated mass of spindle-shaped and stellate cells set in a basophilic mucoid matrix. The tumour is single or multiple and may be bilateral. It is found in as many as 70% of patients with the Carney complex.

11.1.4 Ectopic lacrimal gland

12   Secondary Tumours

Tumours of the Conjunctiva and Caruncle

The caruncle contains elements of the eyelid skin and accessory lacrimal tissue in addition to conjunctival tissue. Benign and malignant entities, both non-pigmented and pigmented, of eyelid, conjunctiva or lacrimal tissue may involve this anatomic site.

1   Epithelial Tumours

1.1   Benign
1.1.1   Squamous cell papilloma (Figs. 12, 13)
Conjunctival epithelium with numerous goblet cells and mucous glands covers a fibrovascular stalk. Papillomas of the infective type are multiple, may be sessile or pedunculated and are found on the lid margins, lacrimal caruncle or limbus, but the most common site is the inferior fornix. Children and young adults are affected. Human papillomavirus type 6 has been demonstrated using molecular hybridization techniques.

The limbal papilloma of adults is usually flat with a broad base, single and unilateral. A varying degree of epithelial pleomorphism and dysplasia can occur.

1.1.2   Keratotic plaque
A focally thick keratin and epithelial layer, most common at the limbus. Dyskeratosis is not usually a feature.

1.1.3   Keratoacanthoma

1.1.4   Reactive epithelial hyperplasia
(pseudoepitheliomatous hyperplasia)
The term "reactive epithelial hyperplasia" is preferred, as it is concise and expresses the pathobiology of the process. The epithelium is acanthotic, parakeratotic or hyperkeratotic and is secondary to chronic irritation or adjacent to a neoplasm such as a keratoacanthoma.

1.1.5   Inverted follicular keratosis
Proliferating epithelium without keratinization or inflammation invaginates connective tissue. It occurs in the juxtalimbal area, plica semilunaris, caruncle or tarsal conjunctiva.

1.1.6   Hereditary intraepithelial dyskeratosis (Figs. 14, 15)
An entity that is inherited in an autosomal dominant pattern consisting of bilateral, elevated, horseshoe-shaped dyskeratotic epithelial plaques at the limbus.

Acanthotic, hyperkeratotic and dyskeratotic epithelium at the nasal or temporal limbus is associated with chronic inflammatory cells within the stroma.

Similar lesions may be present in oral mucous membranes. Descendants of an inbred isolate of Caucasian, Native American and African American origin are at risk. The condition is benign. Most cases are found in North Carolina, but the condition may occur elsewhere.

1.1.7   Oncocytoma (Figs. 16, 17)
This lesion often arises in the caruncle or adjacent canthal conjunctiva. It is also known as oxyphil cell adenoma.

Large cells with eosinophilic granular cytoplasm are arranged in nests, cords or sheets and may form glandular or ductular structures. Ultrastructurally, the cytoplasm is laden with mitochondria.

The majority are slow-growing, benign lesions of the caruncle in older individuals.

1.1.8   Junctional naevus
Nests of naevus cells are confined to the lower portion of the epithelium. The entity occurs only in the very young. An identical appearance in the adult is seen with primary acquired melanosis that lacks
atypia.

1.1.9   Compound naevus (Fig. 18)
This is the most common type of naevus of the conjunctiva. Nests of
naevus cells are found in the subepithelial tissues and at the junctional zone. Melanin pigment may or may not be present. Epithelial embryonic inclusion cysts are a common feature. It occurs most commonly on the bulbar conjunctiva of children. Enlargement, which
occurs at the time of puberty, is largely due to growth of the cysts.
Malignant potential is low.

1.1.10   Subepithelial naevus
This is less common than compound and junctional naevi. Nests of
rounded naevus cells lie within the subepithelial tissues.

1.1.11   Spitz naevus (epithelioid/spindle cell)
1.1.12   Blue naevus

1.1.13   Primary acquired melanosis *without* atypia (Fig. 19)
Deeply pigmented dendritic or small polygonal melanocytes are
present throughout the epithelium. Atypical melanocytes within the
basal layer are lacking or are minimal. Large epithelioid cells are ab-
sent.

1.1.14   Congenital melanosis
Dendritic melanocytes actually lie within episcleral tissues so that
conjunctiva moves over the lesion, which appears grey. This may be
associated with a diffuse ipsilateral naevus of the uvea. The condition
is most common in Orientals. Occurrence in Occidentals is associated with the development of uveal melanoma.

1.1.15   Cysts
Acquired inclusion epithelial cysts are usually secondary to trauma.
Lymphangiectatic cysts may follow mild inflammation or trauma.

1.2   Precancerous

1.2.1   Actinic keratosis

This entity is a plaque-like lesion occurring at the interpalpebral limbus. The epithelium exhibits acanthosis, keratosis and occasionally parakeratosis. The degree of dysplasia is minimal.

1.2.2   Epithelial dysplasia (conjunctival intraepithelial
        neoplasia, CIN)

This interpalpebral limbal lesion may appear as a white plaque or is gelatinous. The epithelium shows minimal keratinization. Dysplasia does not involve the full thickness of the epithelium.

1.2.3   Primary acquired melanosis *with* atypia (Fig. 20)

Primary acquired melanosis with features of atypia such as basilar hyperplasia, epithelioid cells and mitotic figures has a greater malignant potential than the variant that lacks atypical features. Malignant change may not supervene for as long as 20 years.

1.2.4   Xeroderma pigmentosum

1.3   Malignant

1.3.1   Carcinoma in situ (Fig. 21)

This occurs at the limbus. Characteristically, there is a sharp line of demarcation between normal and dysplastic epithelium. Dysplastic cells occupy the full epithelial thickness. Mitotic figures may be numerous. Recurrence is common. Transition to invasive carcinoma is rare.

1.3.2   Squamous cell carcinoma (Fig. 22)

This arises in the exposed interpalpebral limbal conjunctiva of elderly patients. In African and Latin American countries, the tumour occurs in a younger age-group. Growth is usually slow and exophytic. There is usually good differentiation with surface keratinization. Invasion is only superficial, and the course is indolent with little tendency to invade the eye or to metastasize. Histologically, most lesions are well-differentiated squamous cells with keratin formation.

1.3.3   Spindle cell carcinoma

This rare variant of squamous cell carcinoma may behave aggressively. Hyperchromatic, pleomorphic spindle-shaped cells are characteristically located in the superficial layers of the thickened epithelium.

1.3.4   Mucoepidermoid carcinoma (Figs. 23, 24)

This is a rare tumour of the elderly that arises in the perilimbal conjunctiva, most commonly in the nasal area. It is highly aggressive. Histologically, it is composed of an admixture of squamous and mucus-secreting cells. The latter cells may exist in only small foci and may not be apparent until the tumour recurs and/or has invaded the eye.

1.3.5   Malignant melanoma arising in junctional naevi

A history of a long-standing conjunctival lesion, usually pigmented, exists. Histologically, the epithelium that is adjacent to the invading melanoma cells shows the features of the original naevus.

1.3.6   Malignant melanoma arising in primary acquired melanosis *with* atypia (Fig. 25)

1.3.7   Malignant melanoma arising de novo

The clinical and histological features of a pre-existing naevus or atypical melanosis are lacking. Histologically, there is radial growth but no horizontal intraepithelial growth, so that the lesion appears nodular.

2   Lymphocytic Infiltrates

2.1   *Benign (Fig. 26)*

The majority of lymphoid infiltrates are benign. Reactive lymphocytic hyperplasia is a common response to a variety of stimuli that include viruses, bacteria and protozoal infections as well as a response to allergens. Proliferating lymphoid follicles, when present, are regularly spaced, confined to the substantia propria and have mitotically active germinal centres. The deep margin of the lesion is distinct. The infiltrate is occasionally diffuse without follicle formation; the deep margin of the infiltrate remains distinct.

2.2   *Malignant (Figs. 27, 28)*

3   Soft Tissue Tumours

3.1   *Benign*
3.1.1   Pinguecula
A focus of elastic degeneration of the collagen within the substantia propria of the bulbar conjunctiva. A variable amount of telangiectasia may be present.

The lesion appears as a yellowish mass most often located nasally in the exposed interpalpebral area.

3.1.2   Pterygium
A lesion similar to pinguecula, also arising at the limbus and extending onto the cornea.

3.1.3   Keloid
3.1.4   Juvenile xanthogranuloma (Figs. 29, 30)
3.1.5   Fibrous histiocytoma
3.1.6   Myxoma
3.1.7   Telangiectasia
3.1.8   Haemangioma
3.1.9   Lymphangioma
3.1.10 Neurofibroma, localized/diffuse
3.1.11 Schwannoma
3.1.12 Others, e.g. amyloid deposits

3.2   *Malignant*
3.2.1   Kaposi sarcoma
3.2.2   Rhabdomyosarcoma
3.2.3   Malignant haemangioendothelioma
3.2.4   Others, e.g. lymphoma

4   Hamartomas and Choristomas

4.1.1   Dermoid
A noncystic hamartomatous developmental malformation that occurs at the limbus.

Histologically, thinly keratinized squamous epithelium that lacks rete ridges covers dense collagenous stroma containing skin appendages. Bilateral limbal dermoids may be seen in Goldhar syndrome and mandibulofacial dysostosis.

4.1.2   Dermolipoma

A choristomatous malformation that consists of fatty tissue in addition to dermal elements.

The location is usually near the lateral canthus. It may extend between the muscles of the superior complex.

4.1.3   Osteoma

A choristomatous lesion composed of a plaque of mature bone.

It is located in the subconjunctival tissue of the upper temporal quadrant.

4.1.4   Complex choristoma (Fig. 31)

A choristoma that is composed of a variable combination of ectopic tissue such as cartilage, smooth muscle and lacrimal gland. The last predominates.

The lesion is usually unilateral and located in the upper outer quadrant.

5   Secondary Tumours

Tumours of the Uvea

The uvea is composed of the iris, ciliary body and choroid.

The nevi of each component in the uveal tract are similar in their histologic appearance. Those of the choroid tend to be larger than those of the iris and ciliary body. Nevi of the iris are single, nodular or diffuse. Most uveal naevi are composed of one or more of the following cell types:

*   Polyhedral cell with a small ovoid nucleus, finely dispersed chromatin and a small nucleolus. The amount of cytoplasm varies. The melanocytoma consists of large, heavily pigmented polygonal cells of this type (Figs. 32, 33).
*   Spindle cells have elongated nuclei in which the chromatin is dispersed uniformly (Fig. 34)
*   Spindle A cell has a thin, elongated nucleus with an elongated chromatin bar. The nucleolus is indistinct (Fig. 35).
*   Dendritic cell is plump with elongated processes and larger, prominent nucleoli (Figs. 35).

- Balloon cell is rounded with a lightly pigmented, vacuolated cytoplasm (Fig. 36).

Nevi greatly outnumber melanomas.

The commonest malignant tumour is a metastasis to the posterior choroid from the lung or breast. The most common primary malignant tumour of the eye in adults is the malignant melanoma, the most common site of which is the choroid.

The melanomas of each component of the uveal tract are similar in histological appearance. The United States Armed Forces Institute of Pathology (AFIP) modification of the Callender classification is the most reliable prognostic indicator. The size of the nucleolus, rather than the size of the nucleus or shape of the cell, is the most important prognostic feature:

- Spindle B cell is slightly larger than spindle A but also has an elongated nucleus in which the nucleolus is distinct and eosinophilic. The chromatin is coarser than in spindle A (Fig. 37).
- Epithelioid cell has a rounded nucleus with a large nucleolus. The size and shape of the cell varies (Fig. 38).

A large tumour may show such extensive necrosis that it is not possible to subtype the tumour; this is then referred to as a "necrotic melanoma".

Important prognostic features, in addition to nucleolar size, include whole tumour size and extent, vascular pattern, mitotic activity and degree of lymphocytic infiltration.

Melanoma of the uveal tract is most common in white patients and rare in those who are racially pigmented. The majority of patients present in the sixth and seventh decade of life. It is more common in men than in women. Predisposing factors include congenital melanosis, naevi and neurofibromatosis.

1   Tumours of the Iris

1.1   *Benign*
1.1.1   Lisch nodule (Figs. 39, 40)
A hamartomatous nodule, composed entirely of melanocytic cells, usually multiple, occurring in as many as 70% of patients with neurofibromatosis type I.

1.1.2   Melanocytic naevus

1.1.3   Melanocytoma (magnocellular naevus) (Figs. 32,33)
A benign nevus composed of polyhedral cells that have abundant, heavily pigmented cytoplasm and uniform nuclei. Nucleoli may or may not be present.

1.1.4   Ocular melanosis
A congenital hyperpigmentation of the uveal tract with increased numbers of normal melanocytes. Heavily pigmented cells are also present in the episclera.
The condition is usually unilateral and most common in Orientals.

1.1.5   Oculodermal melanosis (Naevus of Ota)
A congenital ocular melanosis associated with congenital hyperpigmentation of the skin in the distribution of the ophthalmic and maxillary divisions of the trigeminal nerve.
Melanocytes are increased in number in the upper dermis in addition to being distributed diffusely throughout the whole of the uveal tract.

1.1.6   Mesectodermal leiomyoma (see ciliary body, Sect. 2.1.7)
1.1.7   Haemangiopericytoma

1.1.8   Histiocytic tumours (including juvenile xanthogranuloma)
Juvenile xanthogranuloma has a mixed component of histiocytes, lymphocytes, eosinophils and multinucleated giant cells of the Touton type. Ocular involvement, of which the iris is the commonest site, includes the ciliary body, cornea, conjunctiva, eyelids and orbit. This entity has been observed in association with neurofibromatosis and Niemann-Pick disease.

1.1.9   Pigmented epithelial cyst
1.1.10   Non-pigmented epithelial cyst (implantation cyst)
1.1.11   Ectopic lacrimal gland
1.1.12   Others, e.g. leiomyoma

1.2   Malignant
1.2.1   Spindle B cell melanoma
1.2.2   Epithelioid melanoma

1.2.3   Mixed melanoma (spindle B cells and epithelioid cells)
1.2.4   Leukemic infiltrates
1.2.5   Medulloepithelioma (extension from ciliary body;
        see ciliary body, Sect. 2.1.8)
1.2.6   Rhabdomyosarcoma
1.2.7   Secondary tumours

2   Tumours of the Ciliary Body

2.1   *Benign*
2.1.1   Melanocytic naevus
2.1.2   Adenomatous hyperplasia (Fuchs adenoma)
2.1.3   Melanocytoma (magnocellular naevus; see iris,
        Sect. 1.1.3)
2.1.4   Reactive hyperplasia of non-pigmented and/or pigmented
        epithelium
2.1.5   Adenoma of the pigmented and non-pigmented
        epithelium
2.1.6   Ectopic lacrimal gland (Figs. 41, 42)

2.1.7   Mesectodermal leiomyoma (Figs. 43–45)
A rare benign tumour composed of cells with both myogenic and neu-rogenic features.

Interlacing bands of elongated, spindle-shaped smooth muscle cells with oval nuclei are arranged in a palisade pattern. The cyto-plasm appears granular and eosinophilic. Positive immunostaining is obtained with muscle-specific actin and S-100.

This tumour is more commonly located in the ciliary body, but may also rise from the pupillary muscle of the iris or within the chor-oid.

2.1.8   Medulloepithelioma (dictyoma) (Figs. 46–50)
An embryonic tumour of the non-pigmented epithelium. Teratoid and non-teratoid forms occur, and either form may be benign or malig-nant.

2.1.8.1 Medulloepithelioma, non-teratoid

2.1.8.2 Medulloepithelioma, teratoid
The histology resembles that of the medullary epithelium; rosettes and small cords of neuroepithelial cells are separated by cystic spac-

es that contain hyaluronic acid. Teratoid variants contain cartilage and, less commonly, glial tissue and/or skeletal muscle.

The tumour may arise in the iris, ciliary body or retinal or optic disk head. The ciliary body is the most common site. The mean age of presentation is 5 years of age.

2.1.9   Neurofibroma
2.1.10 Neurofibromatosis
2.1.11 Schwannoma
2.1.12 Ectopic lacrimal gland
2.1.13 Glioneuroma

2.2   *Malignant*
2.2.1   Spindle B cell melanoma
2.2.2   Epithelioid melanoma
2.2.3   Mixed melanoma (spindle B cells and epithelioid cells)
2.2.4   Necrotic melanoma
2.2.5   Medulloepithelioma, non-teratoid
2.2.6   Medulloepithelioma, teratoid
2.2.7   Adenocarcinoma
2.2.8   Secondary tumours (Figs. 51–53)

3   Tumours of the Choroid

3.1   *Benign*
3.1.1   Melanocytic naevus
3.1.2   Melanocytoma (magnocellular naevus)
3.1.3   Neurofibromatosis (Figs. 54, 55)
3.1.4   Schwannoma (Figs. 56, 57)
3.1.5   Mesectodermal leiomyoma
3.1.6   Diffuse melanocytic hyperplasia
        (in association with systemic carcinoma) (Figs. 58, 59)
3.1.7   Haemangioma (Fig. 60)
3.1.8   Osteoma

3.2   *Malignant*
3.2.1   Mixed melanoma (spindle B cells and epithelioid cells)
        (Figs. 61, 62)
3.2.2   Epithelioid melanoma
3.2.3   Necrotic melanoma

3.2.4   Leukemic infiltrates
3.2.5   Lymphomatous infiltrates
3.2.6   Secondary tumours

Tumours of the Retina

1   Tumours of the Neurosensory Retina

1.1   Benign
1.1.1   Retinocytoma (Figs. 63, 64)
A rare, benign counterpart of retinoblastoma that is usually small, placoid and situated at the posterior pole.

The tumour is composed of small, benign-appearing cells that exhibit photoreceptor differentiation and fleurettes. Fleurettes consist of a "fleur-de-lys" arrangement of large, club-shaped photoreceptor elements. Retinal blood vessels loop into the mass, and calcification is usually a feature.

Some authorities believe that the retinocytoma, the retinoma and the spontaneously regressed retinoblastoma are different names for the same entity.

1.1.2   Astrocytoma (Fig. 65)
Glial proliferations of the retina are considered to be hamartomas (see Sect. 1.1.8 below).

1.1.3   Massive gliosis of the retina (Figs. 66–68)
A benign, non-neoplastic, reactive proliferation of retinal glial cells.

This occurs in response to a variety of pathological conditions that include trauma, chronic inflammatory processes and retinal vascular disease.

The retina is totally replaced by glial tissue in which abnormal, thick-walled blood vessels are present. Some astrocytes may have abundant, pale eosinophilic cytoplasm. Small foci of calcification may be present.

1.1.4   Focal reactive gliosis (Figs. 69, 70)
A benign, focal or segmental replacement of the retina by glial tissue.

This reactive gliosis occurs secondary to a variety of conditions such as chorioretinitis, secondary chronic retinal detachment and vascular occlusive disease.

1.1.5   Capillary haemangioma
1.1.6   Cavernous haemangioma

1.1.7   Haemangioblastoma (von Hippel) (Figs. 71, 72)
This lesion is similar to the cerebellar haemangioblastoma. It is confined to the retina and is usually small, but may occupy the whole of the retina. It is seen in von Hippel disease.

Stromal cells with vacuolated cytoplasm and inconspicuous nuclei occupy the matrix between multiple small, thin-walled blood vessels. Glycogen may be demonstrated. Glial fibrillary acidic protein (GFAP) expression is shown by the stromal cells.

1.1.8   Hamartoma
A congenital non-neoplastic lesion composed of nodules of mature bipolar and/or fibrillary astrocytes.

The lesion is confined to the retina. Multiple lesions are seen in tuberosclerosis. With growth, a flat lesion becomes dome-shaped and calcified.

1.2   Malignant
1.2.1   Retinoblastoma (Figs. 73–77)
A malignant tumour of neuroblastic cells that arises in any *of the nucleated retinal layers.*

A hyperchromatic nucleus dominates the cell. Typically, mitotic figures are numerous. Ischemic coagulative necrosis is common. Growth may be of the exophytic or endophytic type, but is commonly a combination of both. Seeding of viable tumour cells occurs into the vitreous and anterior chamber.

The tumour arises either as a germinal or somatic mutation. Bilateral tumours may have a germinal mutation which is associated with the hereditary form of the tumour; patients present at a slightly younger age than patients with the somatic mutation or non-hereditary form.

1.2.1.1 Undifferentiated retinoblastoma
A retinoblastoma in which undifferentiated small cells with hyperchromatic nuclei and scanty cytoplasm grow in broad sheets.

Mitotic figures are numerous. Necrosis with dysplastic calcification is a prominent feature. Liberated DNA material from the necrotic tissue is deposited in the walls of vessels.

1.2.1.2 Differentiated retinoblastoma
A retinoblastoma showing photoreceptor differentiation with true rosettes of the Flexner-Wintersteiner type.

The rosette has a central lumen surrounded by a limiting membrane which corresponds to the external limiting membrane of the retina. Into the lumen project abortive elements of the photoreceptor cells. Fleurettes (club-shaped bodies arranged in small groups resembling fleur-de-lys) may also be present.

1.2.1.3 Diffuse retinoblastoma
A retinoblastoma with undifferentiated, small basophilic cells growing diffusely within the retina without producing appreciable thickening.

Seeding may occur into the vitreous and anterior chamber. This is the least common type of retinoblastoma, and presentation is towards the latter part of the first decade of life.

1.2.1.4 Spontaneously regressed retinoblastoma
The presence of foci of non-viable, small basophilic cells with or without evidence of degenerated retinal tissue present within an eye that is usually phthisical with extensive bony metaplasia.

Phthisis usually follows a severe inflammation. The exact mechanism of this process remains unknown.

1.2.1.5 Lymphoma
1.2.1.6 Leukemia
1.2.1.7 Secondary tumours (Fig. 78)

2   Tumours of the Retinal Pigment Epithelium

2.1   Benign
2.1.1   Congenital hypertrophy
Congenital focal lesions of hypertrophy of the retinal pigment epithelium.

The cells are larger than usual and contain large, spherical granules.

2.1.2   Reactive hyperplasia
A reactive process of the retinal pigment epithelium which may undergo atrophy, hypertrophy, hyperplasia, migration and metaplasia.

This is a non-specific response to a variety of pathological processes, including inflammation, neoplasm and degenerative processes.

2.1.3 Adenoma (Figs. 79, 80)
A rare benign, discrete tumour arising from the retinal pigment epithelium.

The histological pattern varies; it may be tubular, papillary or vacuolated. The best differentiated tumours have a mosaic pattern.

2.1.4 Hamartoma (Figs. 81, 82)
A combined hamartoma of the retina and retinal pigment epithelium.

It is composed of disorganized glial tissue with numerous blood vessels and cords and tubules of proliferating retinal pigment epithelial cells which appear elongated and concentric.

The majority of tumours occur in males and are diagnosed in the first two decades of life. Growth may occur with leakage of fluid within the mass, resulting in thickening and contraction of the dysplastic retina.

2.2 *Malignant*
2.2.1 Adenocarcinoma (Figs. 83, 84)
Retinal pigmented epithelial tumours that show anaplasia, pleomorphism and increased mitotic activity with or without local invasion of the choroid and optic nerve.

The biological malignant capacity of this entity is questionable.

2.2.2 Lymphoma (Fig. 85)
Lymphomatous infiltration of the retina is usually a manifestation of microgliomatosis of the brain.

3 Tumours of the Optic Disc

The histology of the benign and the malignant tumours at this site are similar to those of the retina and choroid.

3.1 *Benign*
3.1.1 Astrocytoma
3.1.2 Melanocytoma (magnocellular naevus)
        (see iris, Sect. 1.1.3)
3.1.3 Hyperplasia of the retinal pigment epithelium

3.1.4   Medulloepithelioma, non-teratoid
3.1.5   Medulloepithelioma, teratoid

3.2   *Malignant*
3.2.1   Spindle B melanoma
3.2.2   Epithelioid melanoma
3.2.3   Mixed melanoma (spindle B cells and epithelioid cells)
3.2.4   Medulloepithelioma, non-teratoid
3.2.5   Medulloepithelioma, teratoid
3.2.6   Lymphoid infiltrates
3.2.7   Secondary tumours

Tumours of the Lacrimal Gland

Similarities exist between the tumours that occur in the lacrimal
gland and in the salivary glands.

1   Epithelial Tumours

1.1   *Benign*
1.1.1   Pleomorphic adenoma (benign mixed tumour)
        (Figs. 86, 87)
1.1.2   Others

1.2   *Malignant*
1.2.1   Carcinoma in pleomorphic adenoma
1.2.2   Adenoid cystic carcinoma (Figs. 88–92)
1.2.3   Mucoepidermoid carcinoma
1.2.4   Adenocarcinoma
1.2.5   Others

2   Lymphocytic Infiltrates

2.1.   *Benign*
2.2.   *Malignant*

3   Secondary Tumours

Tumours of the Lacrimal Drainage System

The lacrimal drainage system is composed of the canaliculus, the sac and the nasolacrimal duct. Tumours arising in these structures are extremely rare and are histologically similar to those tumours that arise much more commonly in the nasal passages and paranasal sinuses. The majority of the primary tumours are epithelial, and the majority of these are malignant (the reader is referred to the WHO Classification of Tumours of the Upper Respiratory Tract). Soft tissue tumours at this site are so rare that they are not listed. The WHO soft tissue tumour classification should be utilized.

1   Epithelial Tumours

1.1   Benign
1.1.1   Squamous papilloma
1.1.2   Transitional cell papilloma
1.1.3   Mixed cell papilloma
1.1.4   Pleomorphic adenoma
1.1.5   Mucocele
1.1.6   Oncocytoma

1.2   Malignant
The majority of malignant epithelial tumours arise from pre-existing papillomas. Primary tumours of mesenchymal origin are extremely rare. Secondary tumours that extend into the lacrimal sac reflect the histology of the primary tumour.

1.2.1   Squamous cell carcinoma (Fig. 93, 94)
1.2.2   Transitional cell carcinoma
1.2.3   Adenocarcinoma (Figs. 95, 96)
1.2.4   Oncocytic carcinoma
1.2.5   Mucoepidermoid carcinoma
1.2.6   Adenoid cystic carcinoma
1.2.7   Undifferentiated carcinoma
1.2.8   Secondary tumours

2   Melanogenic Tumours

2.1   Benign
2.1.1   Naevi

2.2   Malignant
2.2.1   Malignant melanoma

3   Lymphocytic Infiltrates

3.1   Benign
3.2   Malignant

4   Cysts and Tumour-Like Lesions

4.1   Benign
Cysts arising from the lining epithelium of the nasal lacrimal duct
system may be secondary to obstruction within the passages.

Dacryocystitis and/or canaliculitis. Chronic inflammation, secondary to obstruction, may result in a mass. Care must be taken to ex-
clude an invasive carcinoma.

Tumours of the Orbit

1   Fibrous Tissue Tumours

1.1   Benign
1.1.1   Fibroma
1.1.2   Nodular fasciitis
1.1.3   Fibromatosis
1.1.4   Fibrous histiocytoma

1.1.5   Solitary fibrous tumour (Figs. 97, 98)
The entity "solitary fibrous tumour" is a tan–grey, well-circumscribed
tumour that arises most commonly in the mesothelium of the pleura,
but also occurs within the orbit. The histological features are identical at both sites. The neoplastic cells are fibrogenic and react with
anti-vimentin and CD34.

1.1.6   Juvenile xanthogranuloma
1.1.7   Necrobiotic xanthogranuloma
1.1.8   Others

1.2   *Malignant*
1.2.1   Fibrosarcoma
1.2.2   Malignant fibrous histiocytoma
1.2.3   Others, e.g. neuroblastoma

2   Lipomatous Tumours

2.1   *Benign*
2.1.1   Lipoma
2.1.2   Lipoblastoma (foetal lipoma)
2.1.3   Pleomorphic lipoma
2.1.4   Spindle cell lipoma
2.1.5   Others

2.2   *Malignant*
2.2.1   Liposarcoma
2.2.2   Myxoid liposarcoma
2.2.3   Pleomorphic liposarcoma
2.2.4   Others

3   Skeletal Muscle Tumours

3.1   *Benign*
3.1.1   Rhabdomyoma

3.2   *Malignant*
3.2.1   Embryonal rhabdomyosarcoma (Figs. 99, 100)
3.2.2   Alveolar rhabdomyosarcoma (Fig. 101)
3.2.3   Others

4   Smooth Muscle Tumours

5   Vascular Tumours

5.1   Benign
5.1.1   Capillary haemangioma
5.1.2   Cavernous haemangioma
5.1.3   Arteriovenous fistula
5.1.4   Lymphangioma
5.1.5   Others, e.g. glomus tumour

6   Neural Tumours

6.1   Benign
6.1.1   Neurofibroma
6.1.2   Schwannoma

6.2   Malignant
6.2.1   Malignant peripheral nerve sheath tumour (MPNST)

7   Bone Tumours

7.1   Benign
7.1.1   Chondroma
7.1.2   Osteoma

7.2   Malignant
7.2.1   Chondrosarcoma (Fig. 102)
7.2.2   Mesenchymal chondrosarcoma
7.2.3   Osteosarcoma

8   Lymphocytic Infiltrates

Benign lymphocytic infiltrates occur in Graves disease, reactive hyperplasia, idiopathic inflammatory disease and a number of other non-neoplastic entities, such as Wegener granulomatosis and sarcoidosis. The overwhelming majority of orbital malignant lymphomas are of the non-Hodgkin type. Most of these are diffuse, intermediate and B cell type. Pending the revised WHO lymphoma classification, the reader is referred to the NCI Working Formulation, the updated Kiel classification or the REAL classification.

9   Miscellaneous Tumours

9.1   *Benign*
9.1.1   Meningioma
9.1.2   Ameloblastoma
9.1.3   Melanocytic neuroectodermal tumour
9.1.4   Mature teratoma

9.2   *Malignant*
9.2.1   Melanoma
9.2.2   Olfactory neuroblastoma
9.2.3   Chordoma
9.2.4   Malignant germ cell tumour

10   Secondary Tumours

11   Unclassified Tumours

12   Tumour-Like Lesions

12.1   *Cysts*
12.2   *Mucocele of paranasal sinus*
12.3   *Hamartoma*
12.4   *Heterotopic brain tissue*
12.5   *Meningocoele*
12.6   *Idiopathic inflammatory disease (pseudo-tumour)*
12.7   *Inflammatory polyp*
12.8   *Infective granuloma*
12.9   *Wegener granuloma*
12.10   *Foreign body granuloma*
12.11   *Cholesterol granuloma*
12.12   *"Myospherulosis"*
12.13   *Necrotizing sialometaplasia*
12.14   *Adenomatoid hyerplasia*
12.15   *Oncocytic metaplasia and hyperplasia*
12.16   *Nodular fasciitis*
12.17   *Granuloma pyogenicum*
12.18   *Fibrous dysplasia*
12.19   *Giant cell reparative granuloma*

Tumours of the Optic Nerve

1.1   Benign
1.1.1   Astrocytoma (pilocytic astrocytoma) (Figs. 103–105)
Spindle-shaped astrocytes replace the normal nerve tissue and often
show thickening and distortion of the fibrillary processes (Rosenthal
fibres). Foci of calcification may be present as well as areas of
microcystic degeneration. The tumour cells invade the meninges and
cause a reactive proliferation of the arachnoid elements.

The tumour is slow growing, is most commonly seen in children
in the first decade of life and is associated with neurofibromatosis
type I. It may extend from the optic nerve to the chiasm.

1.1.2   Meningioma (Figs. 106, 107) ·
Primary meningioma of the optic nerve sheath is less common than
orbital meningioma secondary to a primary intracranial meningioma.
The cell of origin is the arachnoid cell, and the tumour is most commonly of the meningotheliomatous type. Those tumours arising near
the optic canal tend to have psammoma bodies.

1.1.3 Melanocytoma (Fig. 108)
Melanocytoma of the optic disk head, also known as magnocellular
naevus is a benign heavily pigmented tumour consisting of uniform
polyhedral melanocytes. It extends from the disk head into the optic
nerve.

1.2   Malignant
1.2.1   Glioblastoma multiforme (high-grade astrocytoma)
             (Figs. 109, 110)
Anaplastic, pleomorphic cells with or without necrosis replace the
normal optic tissue. As a primary tumour it is rare and is found in
adults; more commonly, the tumour is an extension of a frontal lobe
glioma.

1.2.2   Secondary tumours

Metastatic tumours more commonly involve the optic nerve sheaths than the nerve itself. The commonest primary sites are breast and lung.
A secondary orbital meningnoma extends from the cranial cavity and surrounds the optic nerve (Figs. 111, 112)

Phakomatoses (Neurocristopathies)

The word "phakoma" is derived from the Greek word *phakos*, meaning spot or birthmark. The four classical phakomatoses or neurocristopathies are:

1. Neurofibromatosis (von Recklinghausen disease)
2. Tuberous sclerosis (Bourneville disease)
3. Sturge-Weber syndrome (encephalotrigeminal angiomatosis)
4. von Hippel-Lindau disease (retinal angiomatosis)
    Two additional phakomatoses are:
5. Wyburn-Mason syndrome (racemose angioma)
6. Ataxia telangiectasia (Louis-Barr syndrome)

All these entities, with the exception of Sturge-Weber syndrome, are transmitted in an autosomal dominant pattern.

Each phakomatosis (neurocristopathy) has hamartomatous growths of the central nervous system. Hamartomatous growths of the skin may also be present.

1   Neurofibromatosis

1.1   Neurofibromatosis type 1 (NF-1, peripheral neurofibromatosis, von Recklinghausen disease)

The components may include café-au-lait spots, neurofibromas (dermal, subcutaneous, plexiform), Lisch nodules of the iris, choroidal hamartomas, astrocytic tumours of the retina, optic nerve gliomas and a variety of central nervous system (CNS) tumours. Both children and adults are at increased risk for malignant schwannoma.

It is inherited in an autosomal dominant pattern. The NF-1 gene is located on the long arm of chromosome 17 (17q11.2).

1.2   Neurofibromatosis type 2 (NF-2, bilateral acoustic neurofibromatosis, central neurofibromatosis)

The components may include bilateral acoustic neuromas, meningiomas, trigeminal nerve tumours, schwannomas, spinal cord ependymomas and dermal, subcutaneous and plexiform neurofibromas.

It is inherited in an autosomal dominant pattern. The NF-2 gene is located on the long arm of chromosome 22 (22q11.1–22q13.1).

2   Tuberous Sclerosis

The triad of the disease includes: adenoma sebaceum (angiofibromas of the facial skin), epilepsy and mental deficiency.

Components may include angiofibromas (skin), periungual fibromas, café-au-lait spots, subependymal astrocytomas (lateral ventricles), calcified astrocytic hamartomas of the optic disc and cardiac rhabdomyomas.

The disease is inherited in an autosomal dominant pattern, but has low penetrance.

3   Sturge-Weber Syndrome

Facial naevus flammeus is in the distribution of the first and second division of the Vth cranial nerve with or without ipsilateral glaucoma due to angle deformity and/or ipsilateral choroidal haemangioma. It may also include capillary haemangioma (distribution of first and second division of Vth cranial nerve), ipsilateral choroidal haemangioma and meningeal haemangioma of occipital meninges. This disease has no well-defined hereditary pattern.

4   von Hippel-Lindau Disease

All vascular lesions are "haemangioblastomas" and not simply "angiomas". Haemangioblastomas consist of multiple thin-walled vessels between which are foamy or bubbly cells. It is these cells that distinguish the lesion from a simple haemangioma and make a diagnosis of von Hippel-Lindau disease possible. The exact source of the cells is unknown, but some believe they are of glial origin. Sites of occurrence include the retina, cerebellum, brain stem and spinal cord.

This disease has an autosomal dominant pattern of inheritance. The mutant gene has been localized to 3p25–3p26.

5   Wyburn-Mason Syndrome (Racemose Angioma)

Racemose hemangiomas are found in the retina and brain stem. There is no inheritance pattern.

6   Ataxia Telangiectasia (Louis-Barr Syndrome)

Telangiectatic vessels are found in the conjunctiva, cerebellum and skin.

This disease is inherited in an autosomal recessive pattern. The mutant gene has been localized to 11q22–11q23.

TNM Classification of Tumours of the Eye and its Adnexa[1]

Introductory Notes

The following sites are included:

- Eyelid (eyelid melanoma is classified with skin tumours)
- Conjunctiva
- Uvea
- Retina
- Orbit
- Lacrimal gland

Each tumour type is described under the following headings:

- Rules for classification with the procedures for assessing the T, N and M categories
- Anatomical sites where appropriate
- Definition of the regional lymph nodes
- TNM clinical classification
- pTNM pathological classification
- G histopathological grading where applicable
- Stage grouping where applicable
- Summary

---

[1]This text was previously published in Sobin LH, Wittekind Ch. (eds) (1997) TNM classification of malignant tumours, 5th edn. Wiley, New York

Regional Lymph Nodes

The definitions of the N categories for ophthalmic tumours are:

N – Regional Lymph Nodes

NX   Regional lymph nodes cannot be assessed
N0   No regional lymph node metastasis
N1   Regional lymph node metastasis

Distant Metastasis

The definitions of the M categories for ophthalmic tumours are:

M – Distant Metastasis

MX   Presence of distant metastasis cannot be assessed
M0   No distant metastasis
M1   Distant metastasis

The categories M1 and pM1 may be further specified according to the following notation:

Pulmonary	PUL
Bone marrow	MAR
Osseous	OSS
Pleura	PLE
Hepatic	HEP
Peritoneum	PER
Brain	BRA
Adrenals	ADR
Lymph nodes	LYM
Skin	SKI
Other	OTH

Histopathological Grading

The following definitions of the G categories apply to carcinoma of eyelid and conjunctiva and sarcoma of orbit. These are:

G – Histopathological Grading

GX   Grade of differentiation cannot be assessed
G1   Well differentiated
G2   Moderately differentiated

G3   Poorly differentiated
G4   Undifferentiated

R Classification

The absence or presence of residual tumour after treatment may be described by the symbol R. The definitions of the R classification apply to all ophthalmic tumour types. These are:

RX   Presence of residual tumour cannot be assessed
R0   No residual tumour
R1   Microscopic residual tumour
R2   Macroscopic residual tumour

Carcinoma of Eyelid (ICD-O C44.1)

Rules of Classification

There should be histological confirmation of the disease to permit division of cases by histological type, e.g. basal cell, squamous cell and sebaceous carcinoma. Melanoma of the eyelid is classified with skin tumours.

The following are the procedures for assessment of the T, N and M categories:

T categories   Physical examination
N categories   Physical examination
M categories   Physical examination and imaging

Regional Lymph Nodes

The regional lymph nodes are the preauricular, submandibular and cervical lymph nodes.

TNM Clinical Classification

T – Primary Tumour

TX   Primary tumour cannot be assessed
T0   No evidence of primary tumour
Tis   Carcinoma in situ
T1   Tumour of any size, not invading the tarsal plate; or at eyelid margin, 5 mm or less in greatest dimension

T2   Tumour invades tarsal plate; or at eyelid margin, more than 5 mm but not more than 10 mm in greatest dimension

T3   Tumour involves full eyelid thickness; or at eyelid margin, more than 10 mm in greatest dimension

T4   Tumour invades adjacent structures

N – Regional Lymph Nodes

See definitions on p. 36.

M – Distant Metastasis

See definitions on p. 36.

pTNM Pathological Classification

The pT, pN and pM categories correspond to the T, N and M categories.

G Histopathological Grading

See definitions on p. 36.

Stage Grouping

No stage grouping is presently recommended.

Carcinoma of Conjunctiva (ICD-O C69.0)

Rules for Classification

There should be histological confirmation of the disease to permit division of cases by histological type, e.g. mucoepidermoid and squamous cell carcinoma.

The following are the procedures for assessment of the T, N and M categories:

T categories   Physical examination
N categories   Physical examination
M categories   Physical examination and imaging

Regional Lymph Nodes

The regional lymph nodes are the preauricular, submandibular and cervical nodes.

TNM Clinical Classification

T – Primary Tumour

TX   Primary tumour cannot be assessed
T0   No evidence of primary tumour
Tis   Carcinoma in situ
T1   Tumour 5 mm or less in greatest dimension
T2   Tumour more than 5 mm in greatest dimension, without invasion of adjacent structures
T3   Tumour invades adjacent structures, excluding the orbit
T4   Tumour invades the orbit

N – Regional Lymph Nodes

See definitions on p. 36.

M – Distant Metastasis

See definitions p. 36.

pTNM Pathological Classification

The pT, pN and pM categories correspond to the T, N and M categories.

G Histopathological Grading

See definitions on p. 36.

Stage Grouping

No stage grouping is presently recommended.

Malignant Melanoma of Conjunctiva (ICD-O C69.0)

Rules for Classification

The classification applies only to malignant melanoma.

There should be histological confirmation of the disease. The tumour should be distinguished from non-tumourous pigmentation.

The following are the procedures for assessment of T, N and M categories:

T categories	Physical examination
N categories	Physical examination
M categories	Physical examination and imaging

Regional Lymph Nodes

The regional lymph nodes are the preauricular, submandibular and cervical nodes.

TNM Clinical Classification

T – Primary Tumour

TX   Primary tumour cannot be assessed
T0   No evidence of primary tumour
T1   Tumour(s) of bulbar conjunctiva occupying one quadrant or less
T2   Tumour(s) of bulbar conjunctiva occupying more than one quadrant
T3   Tumour(s) of conjunctival fornix and/or palpebral conjunctiva and/or caruncle
T4   Tumour invades the eyelid, cornea and/or orbit

N – Regional Lymph Nodes

See definitions on p. 36.

M – Distant Metastasis

See definitions on p. 36.

pTNM Pathological Classification

pT – Primary Tumour

pTX Primary tumour cannot be assessed
pT0 No evidence of primary tumour
pT1 Tumour(s) of the bulbar conjunctiva occupying one quadrant or less and 2 mm or less in thickness
pT2 Tumour(s) of the bulbar conjunctiva occupying more than one quadrant and 2 mm or less in thickness
pT3 Tumour(s) of the conjunctival fornix and/or palpebral conjunctiva and/or caruncle or tumour of the bulbar conjunctiva more than 2 mm in thickness
pT4 Tumour invades the eyelid, cornea and/or orbit

pN – Regional Lymph Nodes

The pN categories correspond to the N categories.

pM – Distant Metastasis

The pM categories correspond to the M categories.

G Histopathological Grading

GX Grade cannot be assessed
G0 Primary acquired melanosis
G1 Malignant melanoma arising from a naevus
G2 Malignant melanoma arising from primary acquired melanosis
G3 Malignant melanoma arising de novo

Stage Grouping

No stage grouping is presently recommended.

Malignant Melanoma of Uvea (ICD-O C69.3,4)

Rules for Classification

There should be histological confirmation of the disease.

The following are the procedures for assessment of the T, N and M categories:

T categories	Physical examination; additional methods such as fluorescein angiography may enhance the accuracy of appraisal
N categories	Physical examination
M categories	Physical examination and imaging

Regional Lymph Nodes

The regional lymph nodes are the preauricular, submandibular and cervical nodes.

Anatomical Sites

1. Iris (C69.4)
2. Ciliary body (C69.4)
3. Choroid (C69.3)

TNM Clinical Classification

T – Primary Tumour

TX   Primary tumour cannot be assessed
T0   No evidence of primary tumour

Iris
T1   Tumour limited to the iris
T2   Tumour involves one quadrant or less, with invasion into anterior chamber angle
T3   Tumour involves more than one quadrant, with invasion into anterior chamber angle, ciliary body, and/or choroid
T4   Tumour with extraocular extension

Ciliary Body
T1   Tumour limited to the ciliary body
T2   Tumour invades into anterior chamber and/or iris
T3   Tumour invades choroid
T4   Tumour with extraocular extension

Choroid
T1   Tumour 10 mm or less in greatest dimension with an elevation 3 mm or less*

T1a Tumour 7 mm or less in greatest dimension with an elevation 2 mm or less

T1b Tumour more than 7 mm but not more than 10 mm in greatest dimension, with an elevation more than 2 mm but not more than 3 mm

T2   Tumour more than 10 mm but not more than 15 mm in greatest dimension, with an elevation more than 3 mm but not more than 5 mm*

T3   Tumour more than 15 mm in greatest dimension or with an elevation more than 5 mm*

T4   Tumour with extraocular extension

*Note: When dimension and elevation show a difference in classification, the highest category should be used for classification. The tumour base may be estimated in optic disc diameters (dd, average 1 dd=1.5 mm) and the elevation in dioptres (average 3 dioptres=1 mm); other techniques, such as ultrasonography and computerized stereometry, may provide a more accurate measurement.

N – Regional Lymph Nodes

See definitions on p. 36.

M – Distant Metastasis

See definitions on p. 36.

pTNM Pathological Classification

The pT, pN and pM categories correspond to the T, N and M categories.

G Histopathological Grading

GX   Grade cannot be assessed
G1   Spindle cell melanoma
G2   Mixed cell melanoma
G3   Epithelioid cell melanoma

V Venous Invasion

VX   Venous invasion cannot be assessed
V0   Veins do not contain tumour
V1   Veins in melanoma contain tumour
V2   Vortex veins contain tumour

S Scleral Invasion

SX   Scleral invasion cannot be assessed
S0   Sclera does not contain tumour
S1   Intrascleral* invasion of tumour
S2   Extrascleral invasion of tumour

Note: Includes perineural and perivascular invasion of scleral canals.

Stage Grouping

If more than one of the uveal structures is involved, the classification of the most affected structure should be used.

Iris and Ciliary Body

Stage I	T1	N0	M0
Stage II	T2	N0	M0
Stage III	T3	N0	M0
Stage IVA	T4	N0	M0
Stage IVB	Any T	N1	M0
	Any T	Any N	M1

Choroid

Stage IA	T1a	N0	M0
Stage IB	T1b	N0	M0
Stage II	T2	N0	M0
Stage III	T3	N0	M0
Stage IVA	T4	N0	M0
Stage IVB	Any T	N1	M0
	Any T	Any N	M1

Retinoblastoma (ICD-O C69.2)

Rules for Classification

In bilateral cases, each eye should be classified separately. The classification does not apply to complete spontaneous regression of the tumour. There should be histological confirmation of the disease in an enucleated eye.

The following are the procedures for assessment of the T, N and M categories:

T categories   Physical examination and imaging
N categories   Physical examination
M categories   Physical examination and imaging; examination of bone marrow and cerebrospinal fluid may enhance the accuracy of appraisal

Regional Lymph Nodes

The regional lymph nodes are the preauricular, submandibular and cervical nodes.

TNM Clinical Classification

The extent of retinal involvement is indicated as a percentage.

T – Primary Tumour

TX   Primary tumour cannot be assessed
T0   No evidence of primary tumour
T1   Tumour(s) limited to 25% of the retina or less
T2   Tumour(s) involve(s) more than 25% but not more than 50% of the retina
T3   Tumour(s) involve(s) more than 50% of the retina and/or invade(s) beyond the retina but remain(s) intraocular
    T3a Tumour(s) involve(s) more than 50% of the retina and/or tumour cells in the vitreous body
    T3b Tumour(s) involve(s) optic disc
    T3c Tumour(s) involve(s) anterior chamber and/or uvea
T4   Tumour with extraocular invasion
    T4a Tumour invades retrobulbar optic nerve
    T4b Extraocular extension other than invasion of optic nerve

Note: The following suffixes may be added to the appropriate T categories:
(m)   To indicate multiple tumours, e.g. T2(m)
(f)   To indicate cases with a known family history
(d)   To indicate diffuse retinal involvement without the formation of discrete masses

N – Regional Lymph Nodes

See definitions on p. 36.

M – Distant Metastasis

See definitions on p. 36.

pTNM Pathological Classification

pT – Primary Tumour

pTX   Primary tumour cannot be assessed
pT0   No evidence of primary tumour
pTI   Corresponds to TI
pT2   Corresponds to T2
pT3   Corresponds to T3
      pT3a Corresponds to T3a
      pT3b Tumour invades optic nerve as far as lamina cribrosa
      pT3c Tumour in anterior chamber and/or invasion with thickening of uvea and/or intrascleral invasion
pT4   Corresponds to T4
      pT4a Intraneural tumour beyond lamina cribrosa, but not at line of resection
      pT4b Tumour at line of resection or other extraocular extension

pN – Regional Lymph Nodes

The pN categories correspond to the N categories.

pM – Distant Metastasis

The pM categories correspond to the M categories.

Stage Grouping

Stage IA	T1	N0	M0
Stage 1B	T2	N0	M0
Stage IIA	T3a	N0	M0
Stage IIB	T3b	N0	M0
Stage IIC	T3c	N0	M0
Stage IIIA	T4a	N0	M0
Stage IIIB	T4b	N0	M0
Stage IV	Any T	N1	M0
	Any T	Any N	M1

Sarcoma of Orbit (ICD-O C69.6)

Rules for Classification

The classification applies only to sarcomas of soft tissue and bone. There should be histological confirmation of the disease to permit division of cases by histological type.

The following are the procedures for assessment of the T, N and M categories:

T categories   Physical examination and imaging
N categories   Physical examination
M categories   Physical examination and imaging

Regional Lymph Nodes

The regional lymph nodes are the preauricular, submandibular and cervical lymph nodes.

TNM Clinical Classification

T – Primary Tumour

TX   Primary tumour cannot be assessed
T0   No evidence of primary tumour
T1   Tumour 15 mm or less in greatest dimension
T2   Tumour more than 15 mm in greatest dimension
T3   Tumour of any size with diffuse invasion of orbital tissues and/or bony walls
T4   Tumour invades beyond the orbit to adjacent sinuses and/or to cranium

N – Regional Lymph Nodes

See definitions on p. 36.

M – Distant Metastasis

See definitions on p. 36.

pTNM Pathological Classification

The pT, pN and pM categories correspond to the T, N and M categories.

G Histopathological Grading

See definitions on p. 36.

Histopathological grading of the tumour should be reported and may have an effect on the staging of these tumours; however, no stage grouping is presently recommended.

Stage Grouping

No stage grouping is presently recommended.

Carcinoma of Lacrimal Gland (ICD-O C69.5)

Rules for Classification

There should be histological confirmation of the disease to permit division of cases by histological type.

The following are the procedures for assessment of the T, N and M categories:

T categories	Physical examination and imaging
N categories	Physical examination
M categories	Physical examination and imaging

Regional Lymph Nodes

The regional lymph nodes are the preauricular, submandibular and cervical lymph nodes.

TNM Clinical Classification

T – Primary Tumour

TX   Primary tumour cannot be assessed
T0   No evidence of primary tumour
T1   Tumour 2.5 cm or less in greatest dimension, limited to the lacrimal gland
T2   Tumour 2.5 cm or less in greatest dimension, invading the periosteum of the fossa of the lacrimal gland
T3   Tumour more than 2.5 cm but not more than 5 cm in greatest dimension

T3a   Tumour limited to the lacrimal gland
T3b   Tumour invades the periosteum of the fossa of the lacrimal gland
T4   Tumour more than 5 cm in greatest dimension
T4a   Tumour invades orbital soft tissues, optic nerve or globe, but *without* bone invasion
T4b   Tumour invades orbital soft tissues, optic nerve or globe, *with* bone invasion

N – Regional Lymph Nodes

See definitions on p. 36.

M – Distant Metastasis

See definitions on p. 36.

pTNM Pathological Classification

The pT, pN and pM categories correspond to the T, N and M categories.

G Histopathological Grading

GX   Grade of differentiation cannot be assessed
G1   Well differentiated
G2   Moderately differentiated; includes adenoid cystic carcinoma without basaloid (solid) pattern
G3   Poorly differentiated; includes adenoid cystic carcinoma with basaloid (solid) pattern
G4   Undifferentiated

Stage Grouping

No stage grouping is presently recommended.

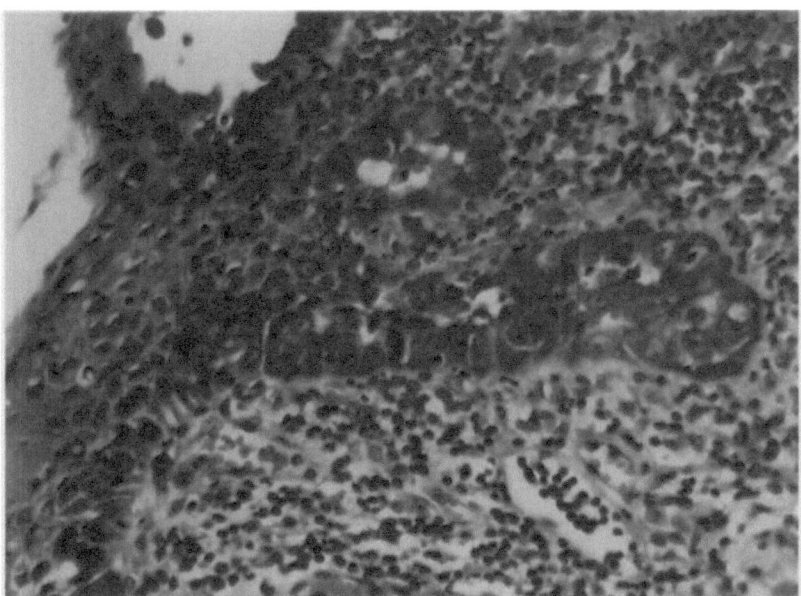

Fig. 1. *Pagetoid changes*, eyelid. Epithelium contains swollen pagetoid cells. Sebaceous adenocarcinoma was present in deep tissue

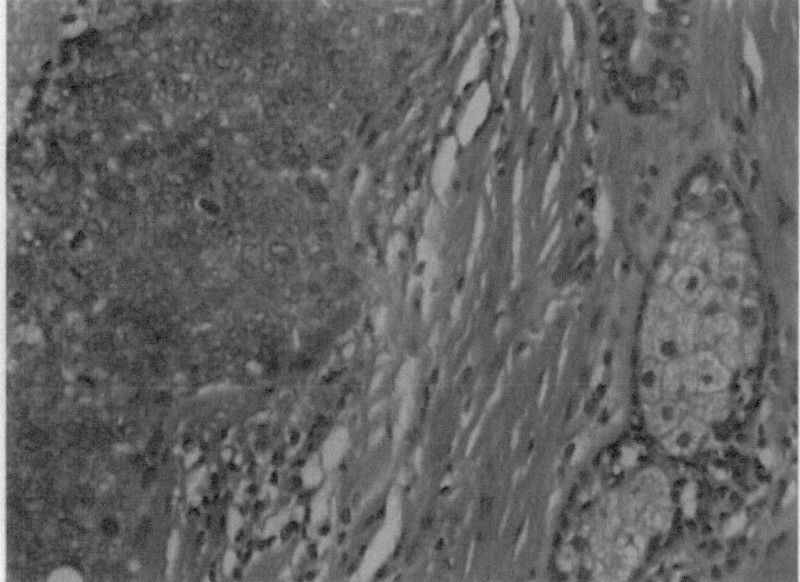

Fig. 2. *Sebaceous cell carcinoma*, eyelid. Undifferentiated sebaceous adenocarcinoma adjacent to normal sebaceous lobule

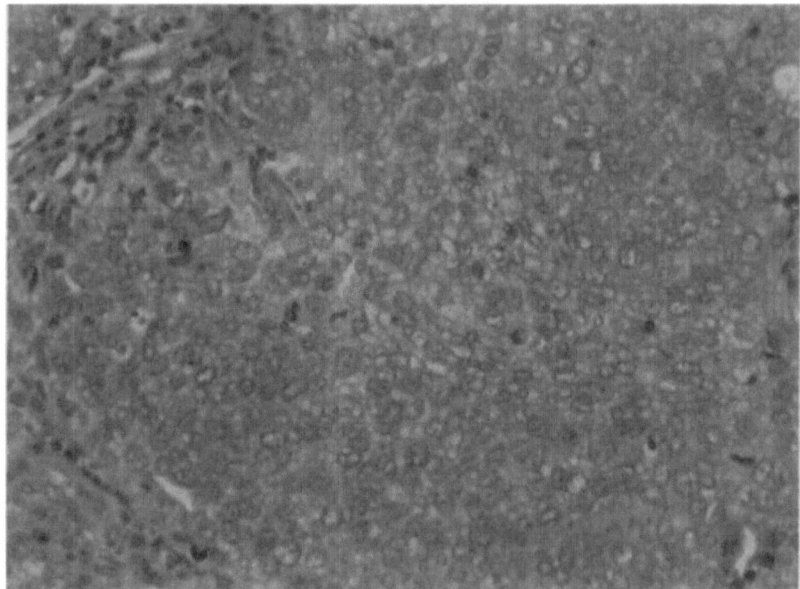

Fig. 3. *Undifferentiated sebaceous cell adenocarcinoma*, eyelid. Nuclei are large and vesicular and have distinct nucleoli. Cytoplasm is foamy

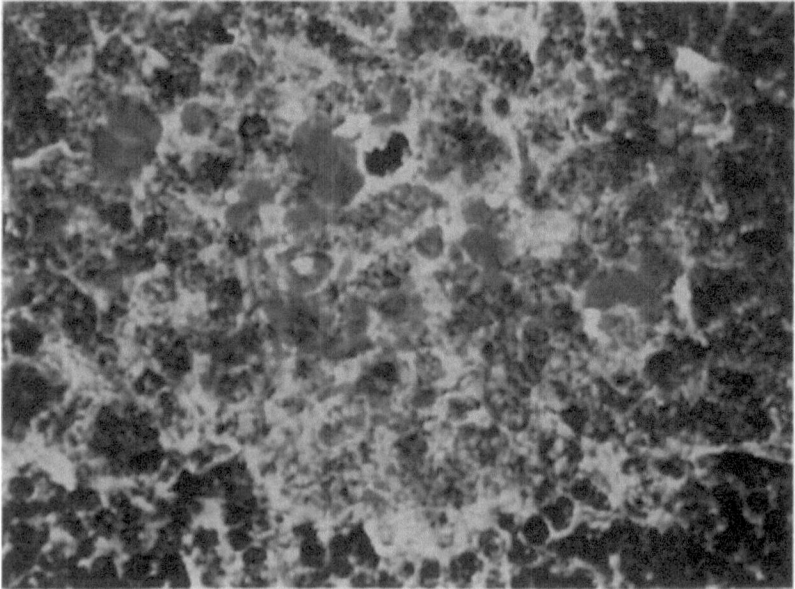

Fig. 4. *Sebaceous cell adenocarcinoma*, eyelid. Oil red-O stain on frozen tissue shows red staining of fat within cytoplasm

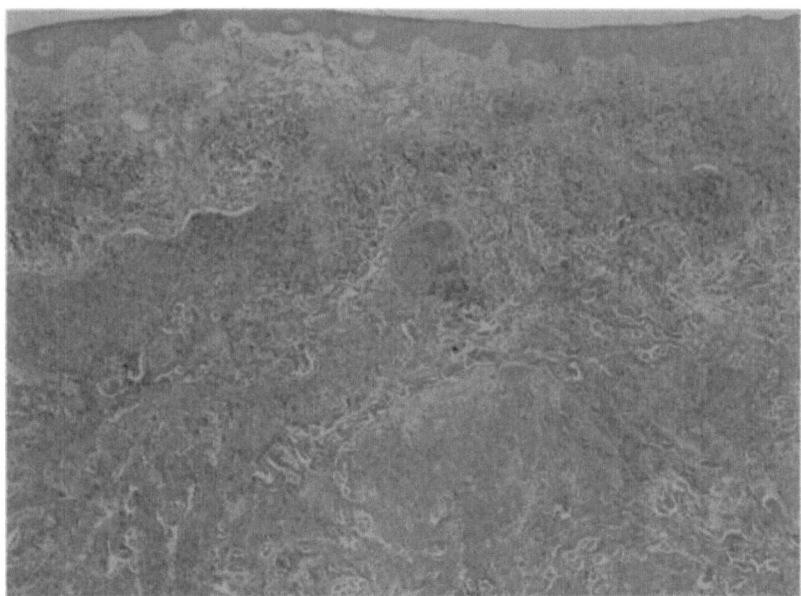

Fig. 5. *Merkel cell tumour*, eyelid. Nests of small dark cells are separated from the epidermis by connective tissue

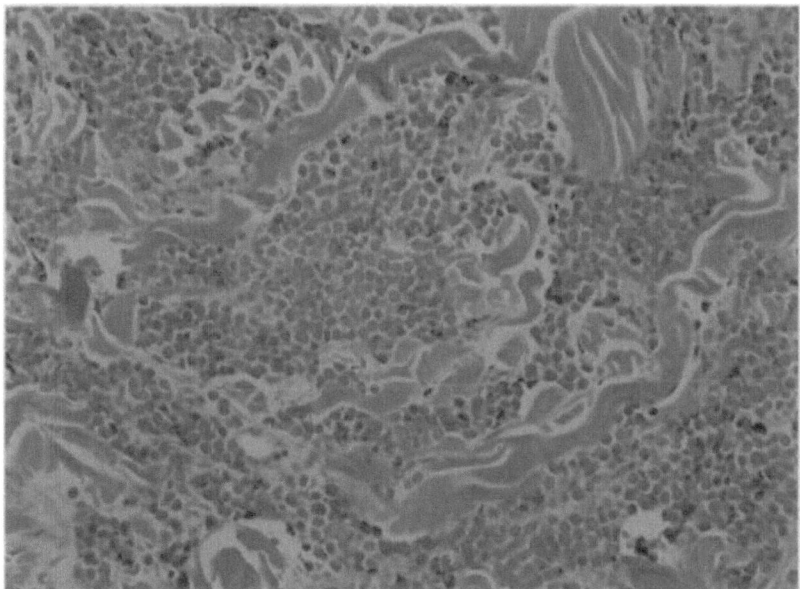

Fig. 6. *Merkel cell tumour*, eyelid. Same tissue as in Fig. 5. Intradermal nests of small, dark, poorly differentiated cells

54

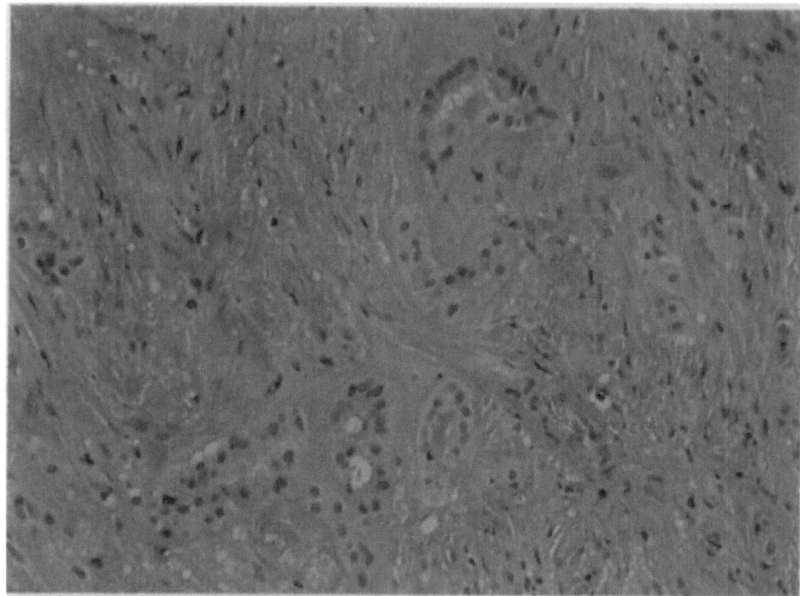

Fig. 7. *Phakomatous choristoma*, lower eyelid. Nests of lens epithelial cells lie in a collagenous matrix

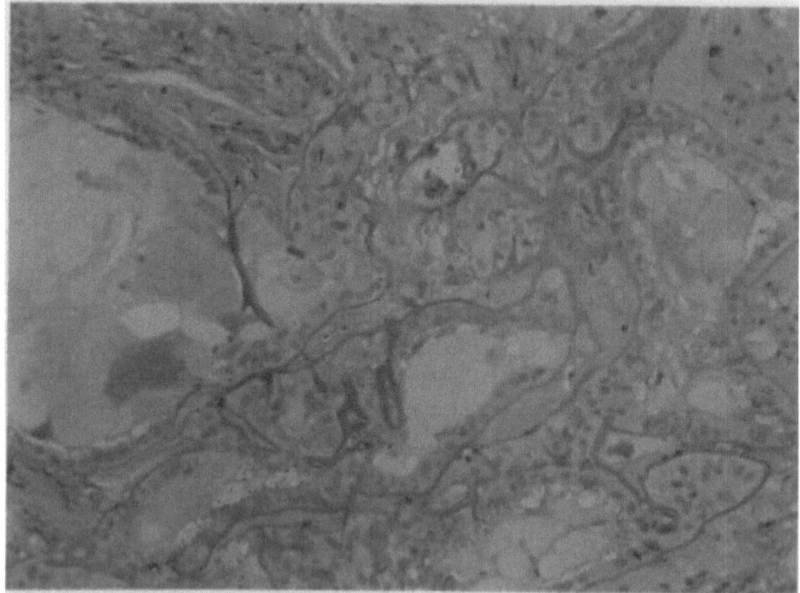

Fig. 8. *Phakomatous choristoma*, lower eyelid. A thick, periodic acid–Schiff (PAS)-positive membrane surrounds a nest of lens epithelial cells

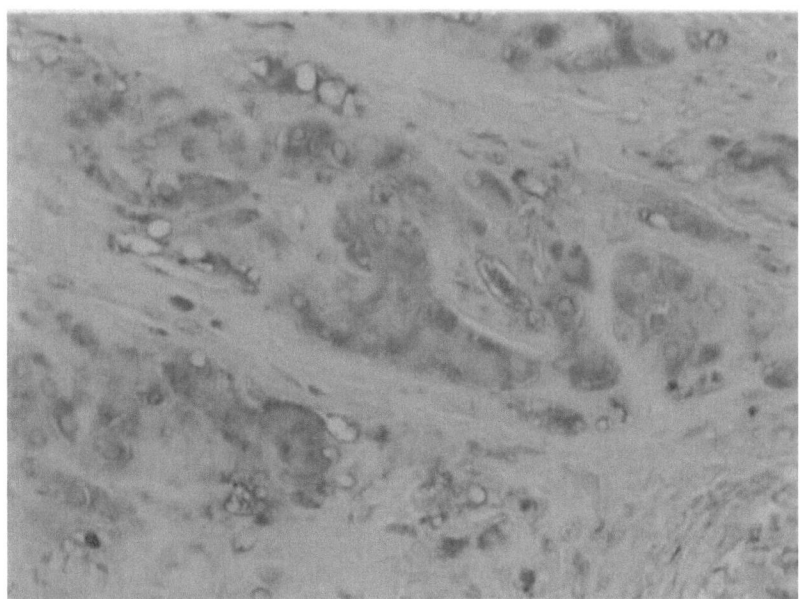

Fig. 9. *Phakomatous choristoma*, lower eyelid. Immunohistochemical stains are positive for anti-alpha crystallin peptide 81

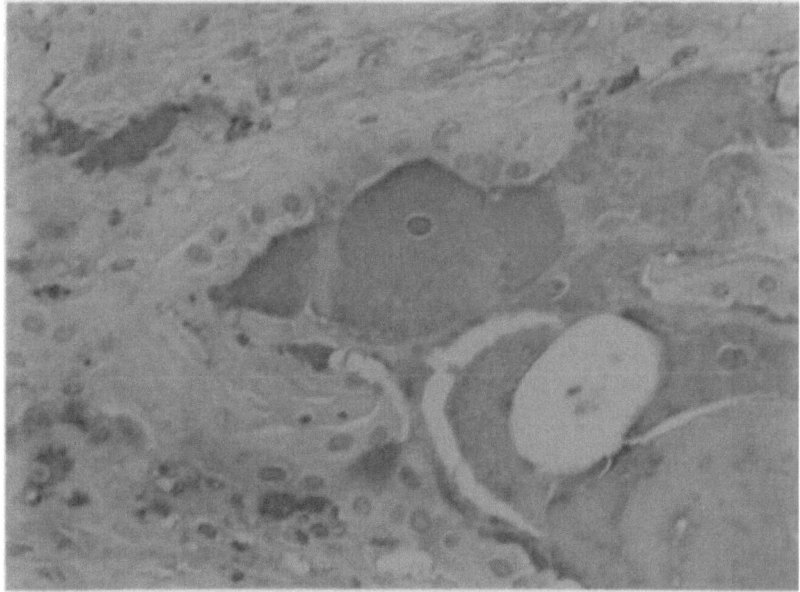

Fig. 10. *Phakomatous choristoma*, lower eyelid. Immunopositivity with anti-beta crystallin

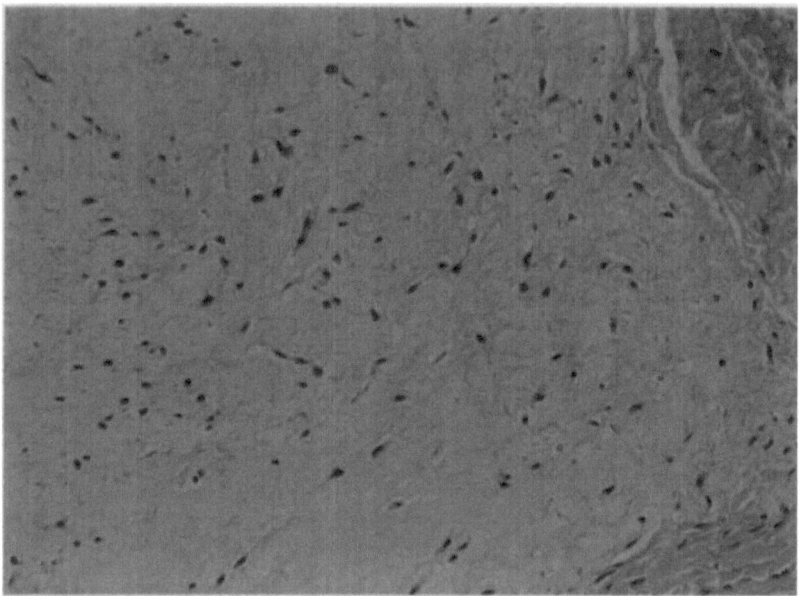

Fig. 11. *Myxoma*, eyelid. Abundant mucoid stroma contains stellate and spindle-shaped cells. Patient also had a myxoma of the heart and facial pigmentation (Carney complex)

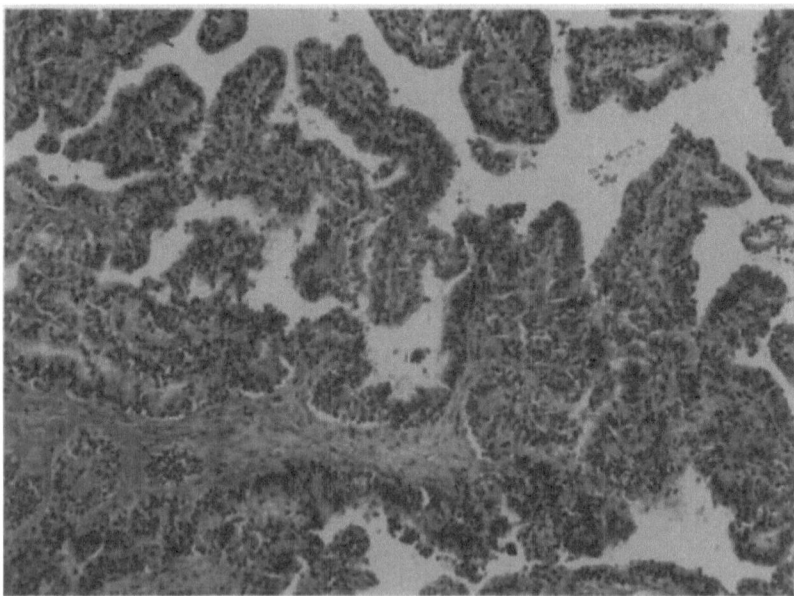

Fig. 12. *Squamous cell papilloma*, conjunctiva. The acanthotic epithelium has many vascular cores

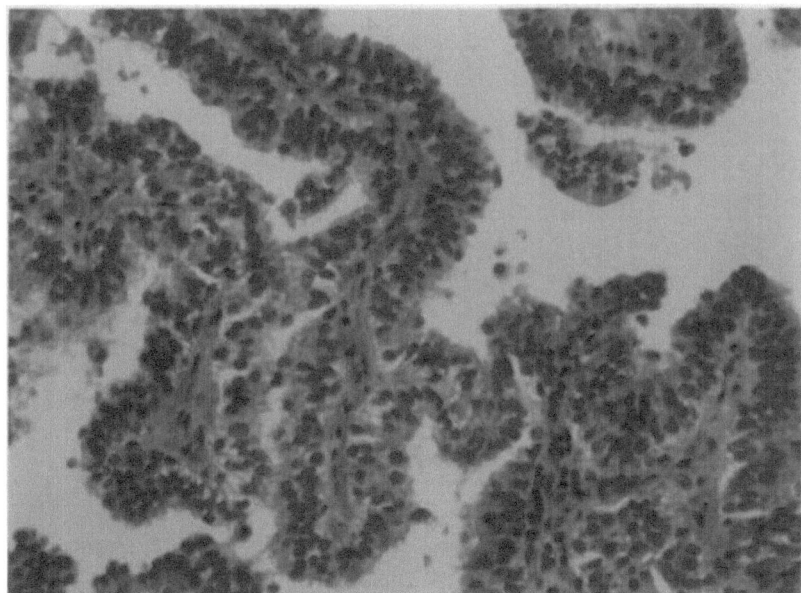

Fig. 13. *Squamous cell papilloma*, conjunctiva. Same tumour as in Fig. 12, showing vascular cores within proliferating epithelial fronds

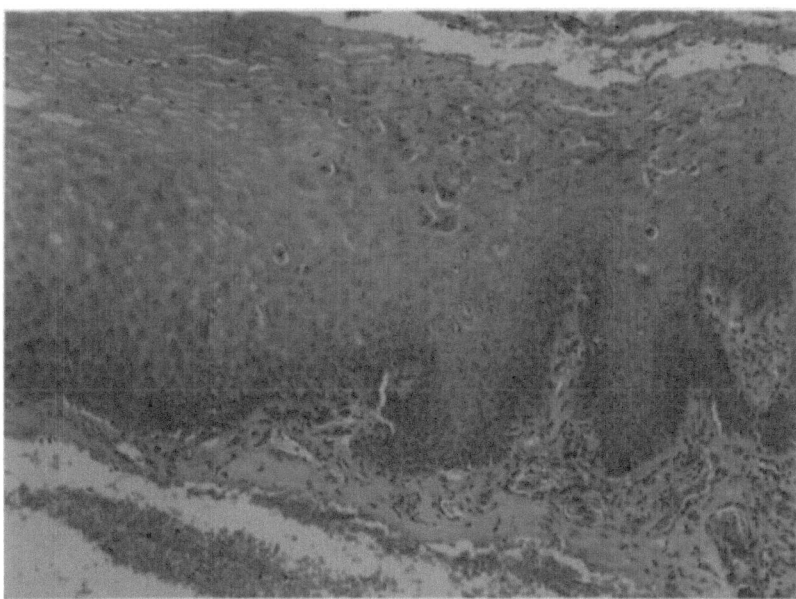

Fig. 14. *Hereditary benign intraepithelial dyskeratosis* (HBID). Lesion from limbus consists of acanthotic epithelium with dyskeratotic cells

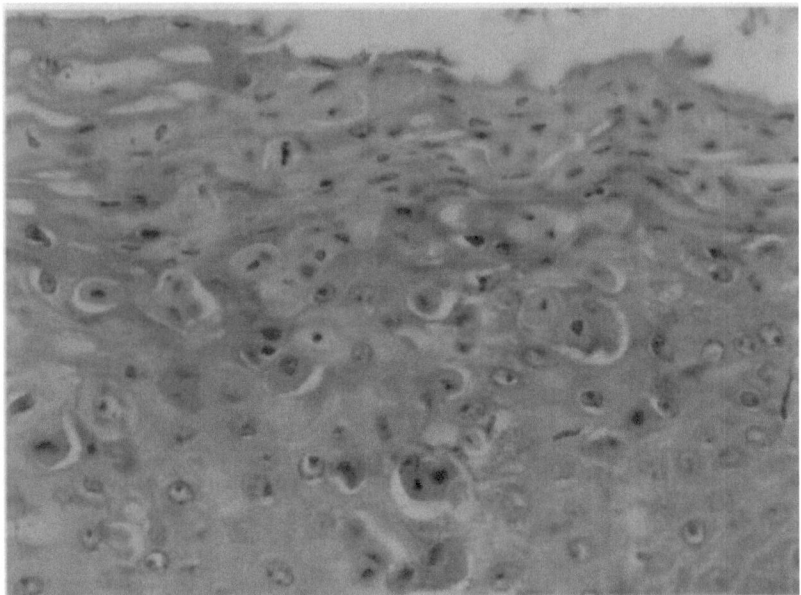

Fig. 15. *Hereditary benign intraepithelial dyskeratosis* (HBID). Same tissue as in Fig. 14 at increased magnification

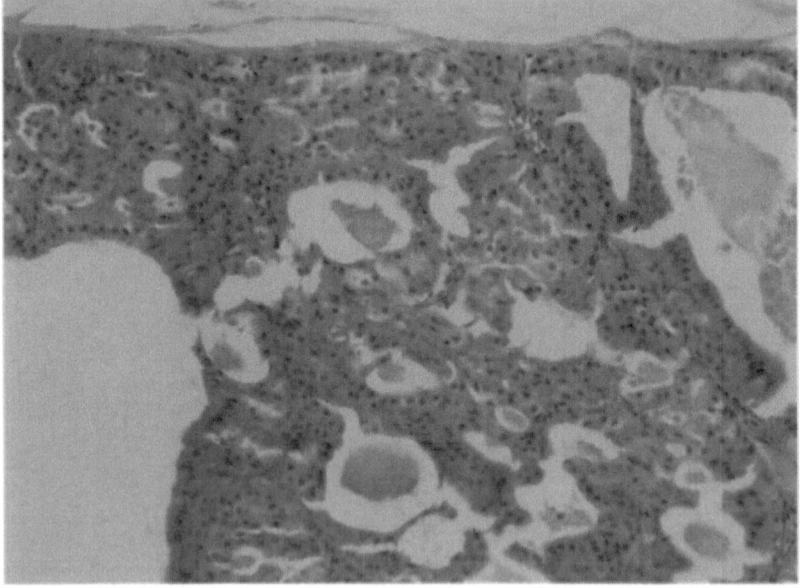

Fig. 16. *Oncocytoma*, caruncle. Epithelial cells with apocrine metaplasia line cystic cavities

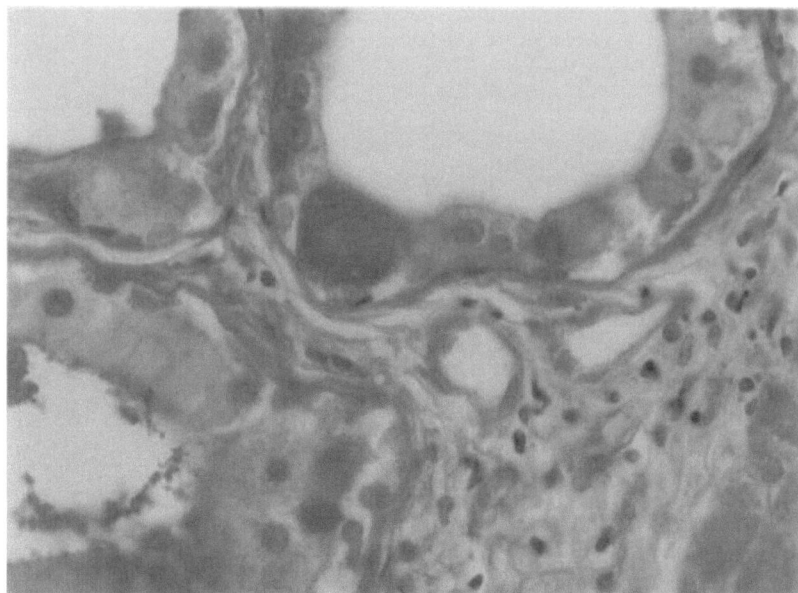

Fig. 17. *Oncocytoma*, caruncle. Same tumour as in Fig. 16 stained with periodic acid–Schiff (PAS). Positive staining of granular cytoplasm reflects abundant mitochondria

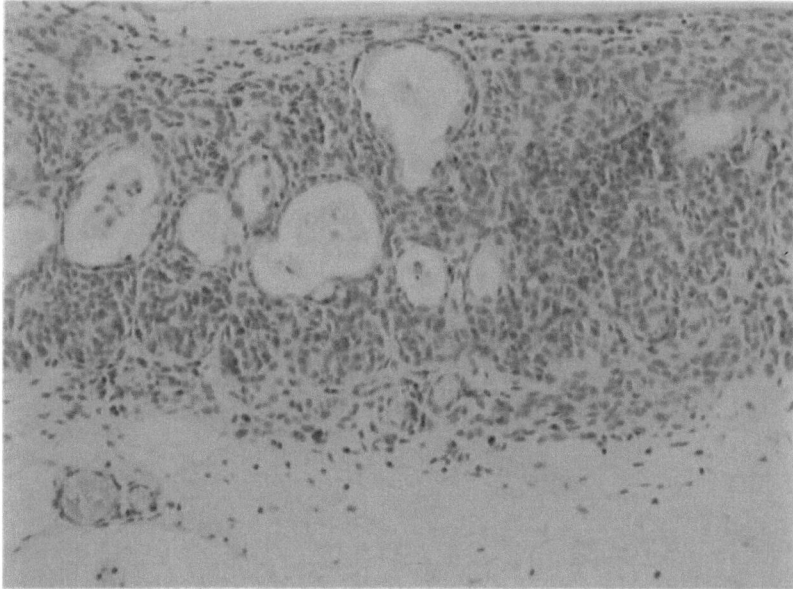

Fig. 18. *Compound naevus*, conjunctiva. Epithelial cysts lined by goblet cells are a common feature

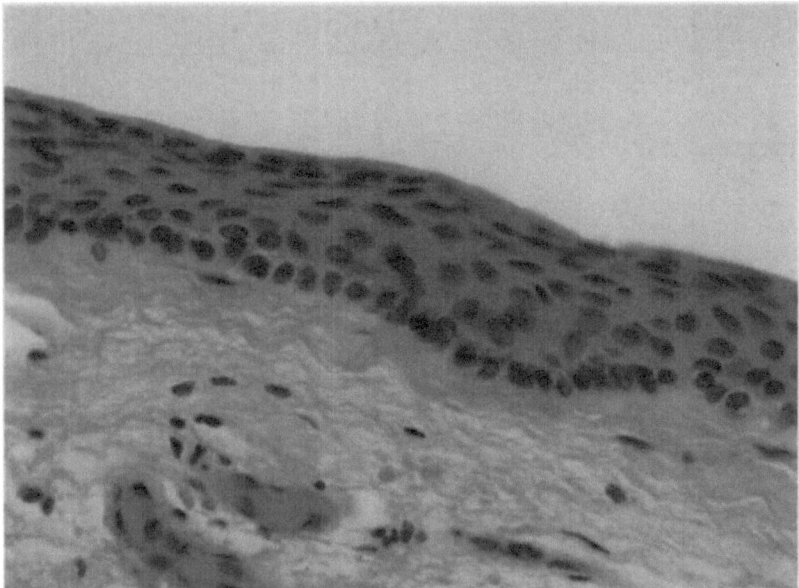

Fig. 19. *Primary acquired melanosis without atypia*, bulbar conjunctiva. Pigmentation is confined to the basal cells. Epithelial cells show maturation

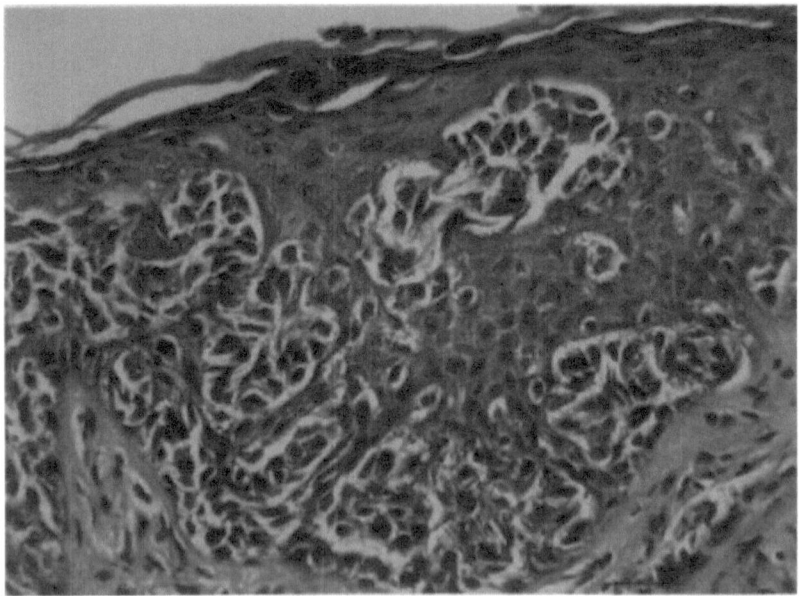

Fig. 20. *Primary acquired melanosis with atypia*, bulbar conjunctiva. Proliferating atypical cells invade the epithelium

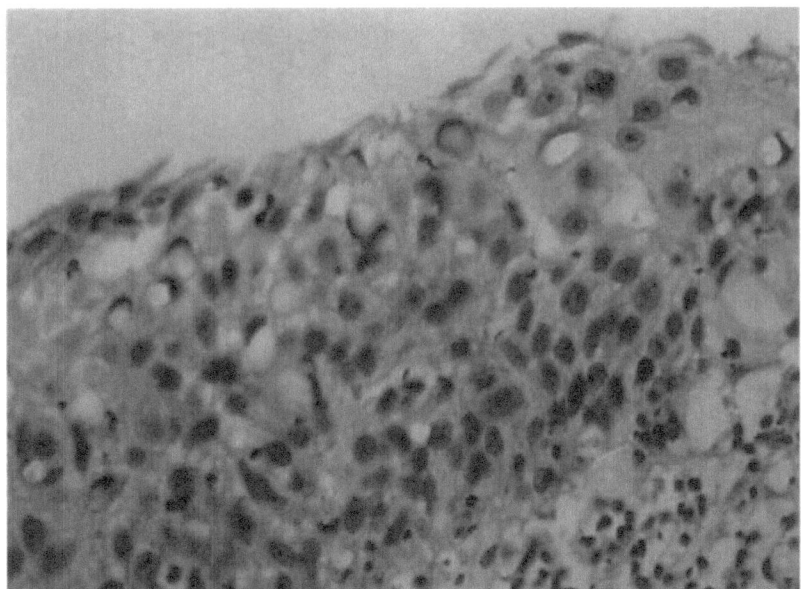

Fig. 21. *Carcinoma in situ*, limbus. Atypical cells occupy full thickness of epithelium

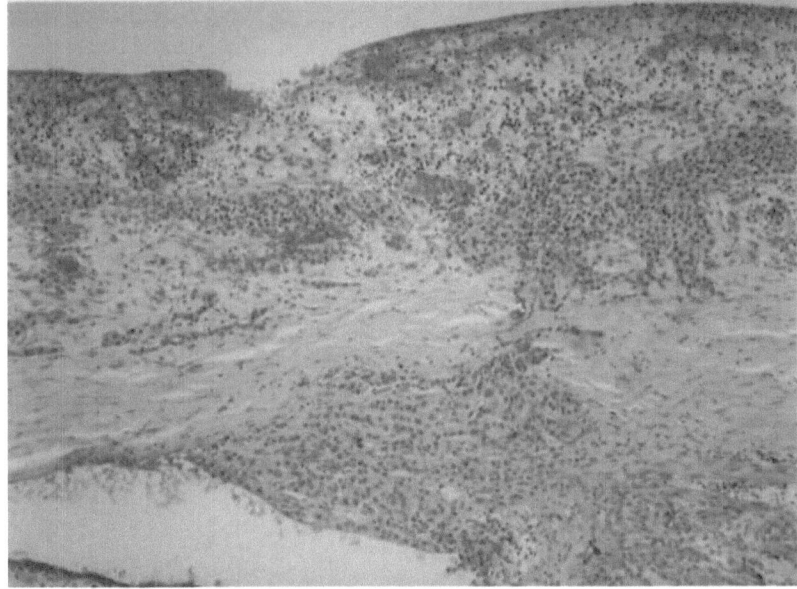

Fig. 22. *Infiltrating squamous cell carcinoma*, limbus. The malignant cells invade the limbal stroma and extend between the corneal lamellae and into the trabecular meshwork

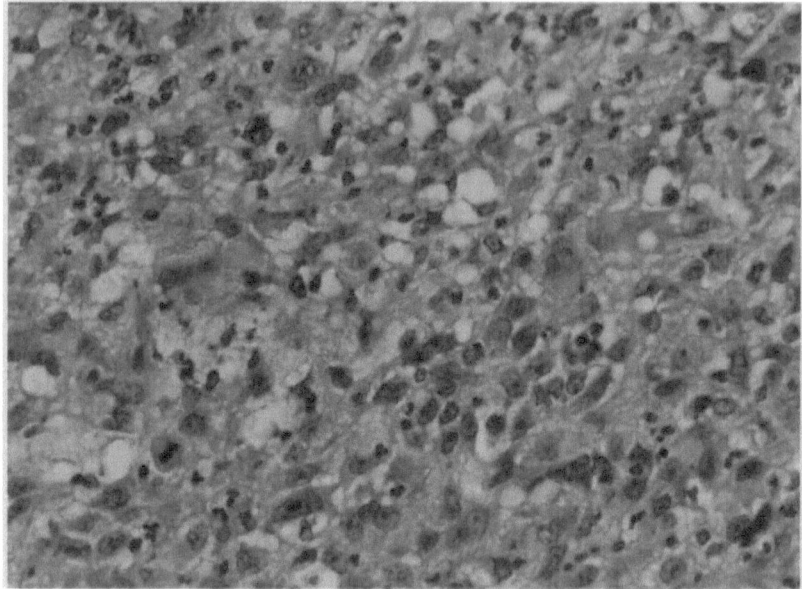

Fig. 23. *Mucoepidermoid carcinoma*, conjunctiva. Exophytic growth pattern

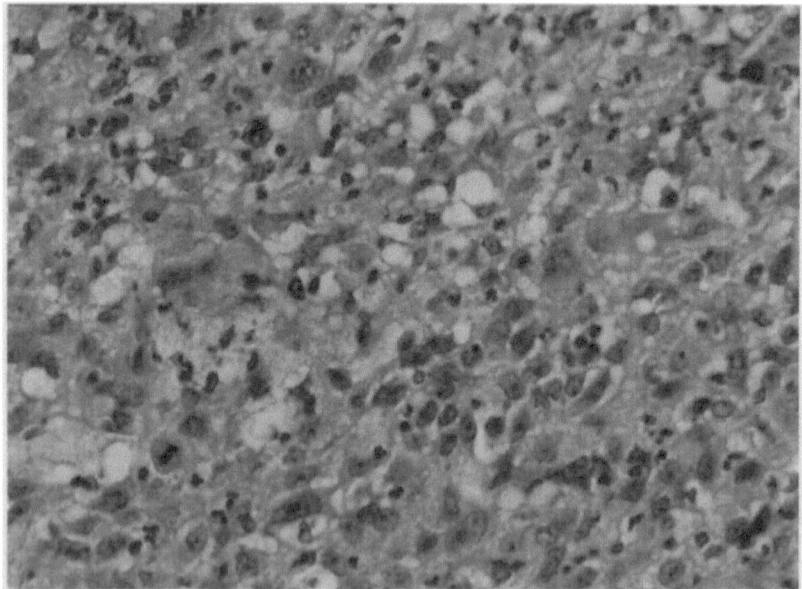

Fig. 24. *Mucoepidermoid carcinoma*, conjunctiva. Undifferentiated tumour with isolated mucus-containing cells showing basophilic staining

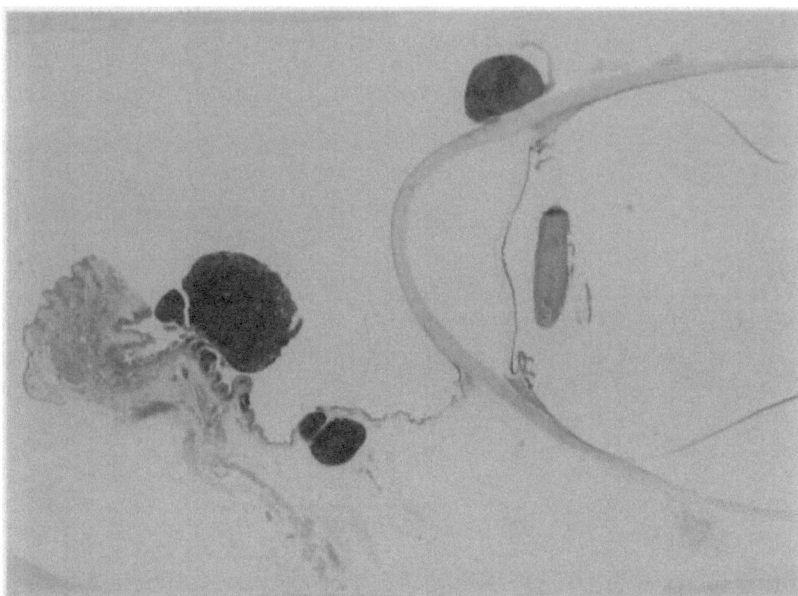

Fig. 25. *Malignant melanoma*, conjunctiva. Multiple foci of malignant melanoma arising in primary acquired melanosis with atypia

Fig. 26. *Reactive lymphocytic hyperplasia*, conjunctiva. Mature follicles show reactive centres

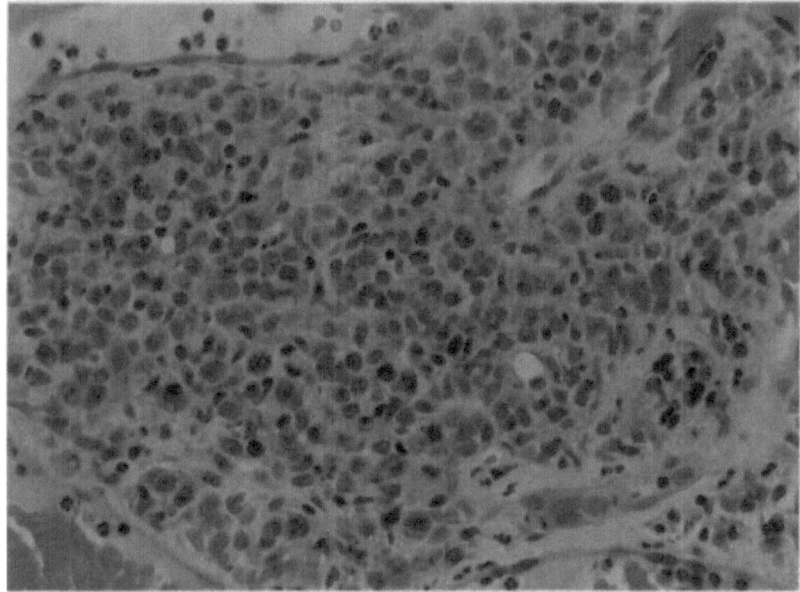

Fig. 27. *Lymphoma*, conjunctiva. Large B-cell type

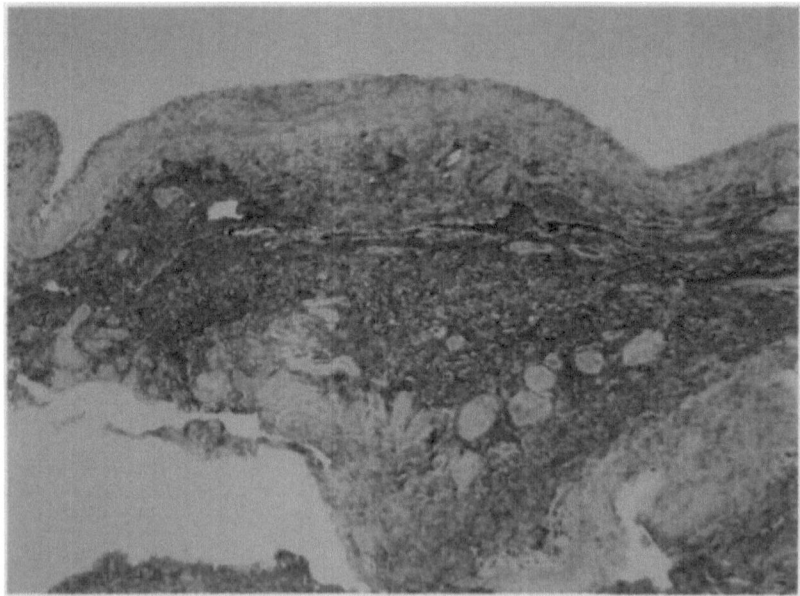

Fig. 28. *Lymphoma*, conjunctiva. Monoclonal kappa staining of large B cell-type lymphoma

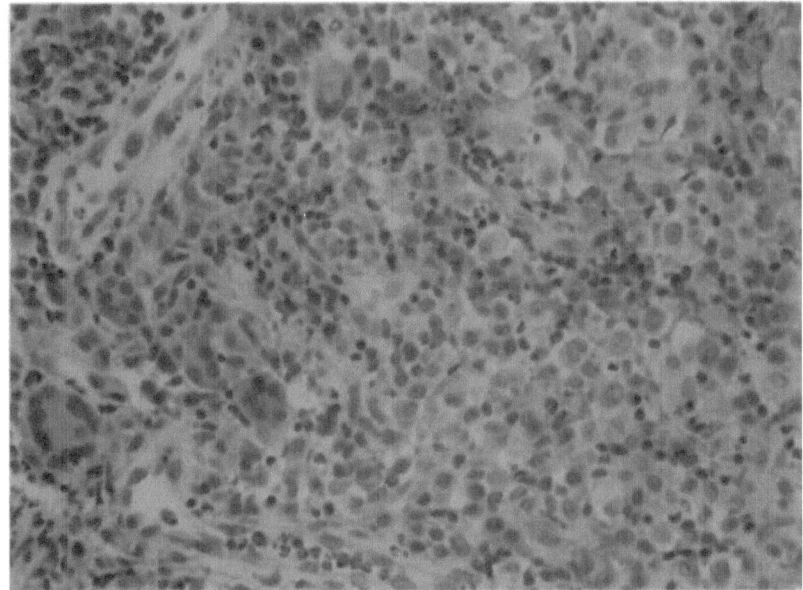

Fig. 29. *Juvenile xanthogranuloma*, conjunctiva. Diffuse infiltration by histiocytes, eosinophils and giant cells

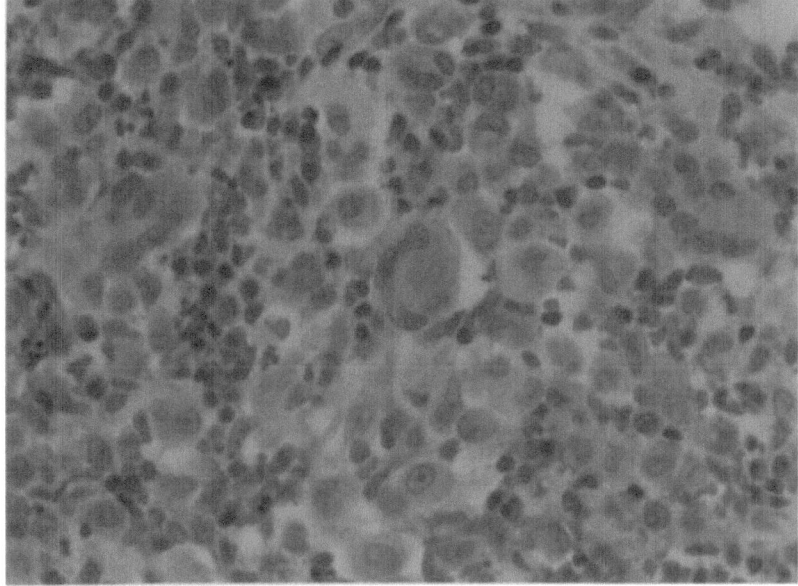

Fig. 30. *Juvenile xanthogranuloma*, conjunctiva. Same tumour as in Fig. 29, showing giant cells of Touton type

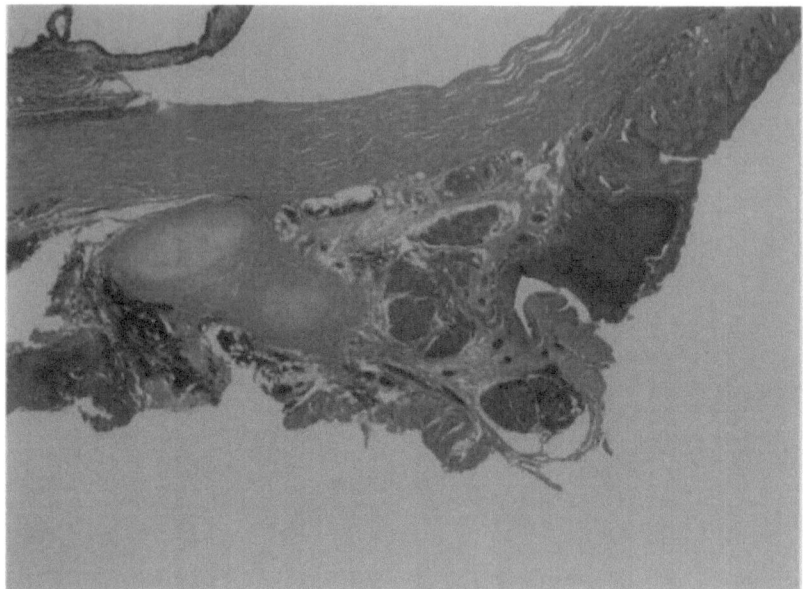

Fig. 31. *Complex choristoma*, limbus. Limbal mass composed of lacrimal tissue and cartilage

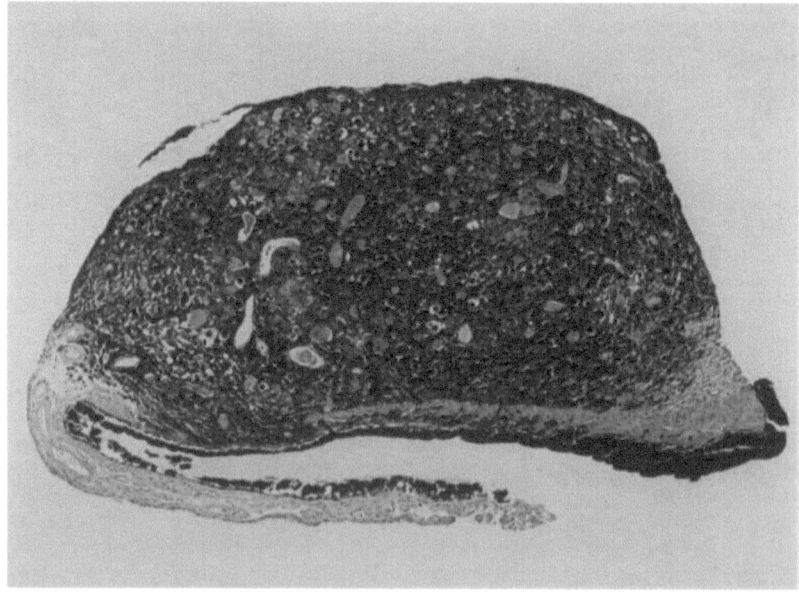

Fig. 32. *Melanocytoma*, iris. Heavily pigmented nodule with prominent iris stromal vessels

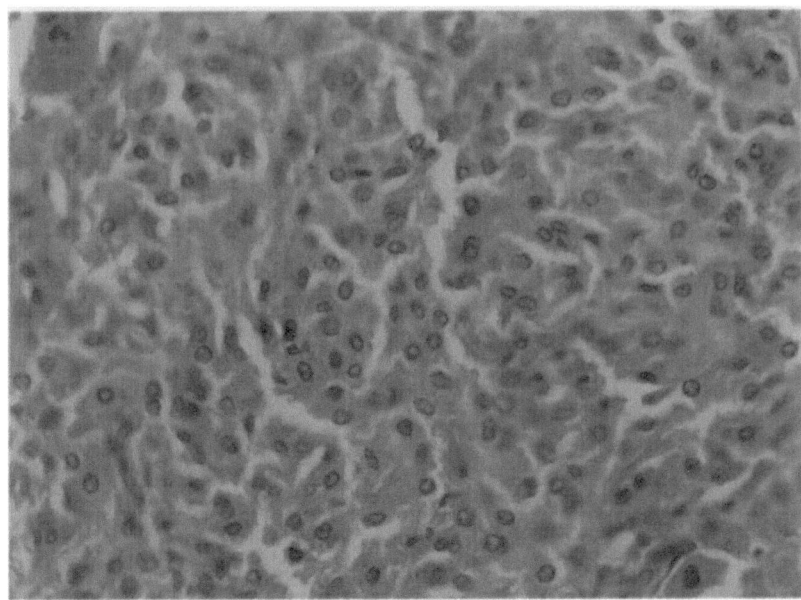

Fig. 33. *Melanocytoma*, iris. Same tumour as in Fig. 32. Bleached section shows uniform polyhedral cells with abundant cytoplasm and well-defined cytoplasmic membrane. A nucleolus is present in occasional cells

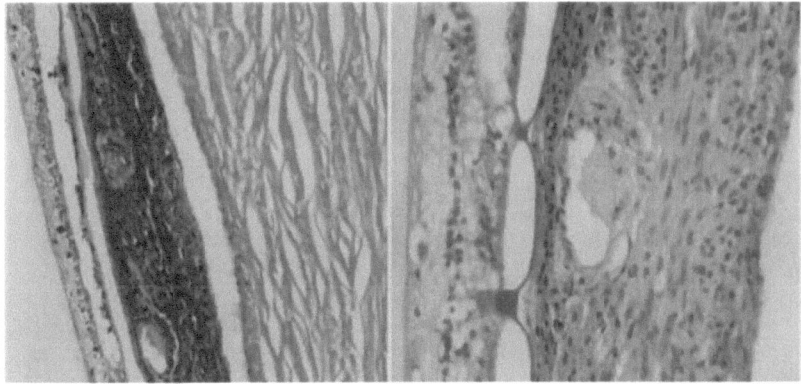

Fig. 34. *Naevus*, choroid. Heavy pigmentation obscures spindle cells (*left*). Bleached section reveals character of nuclei (*right*)

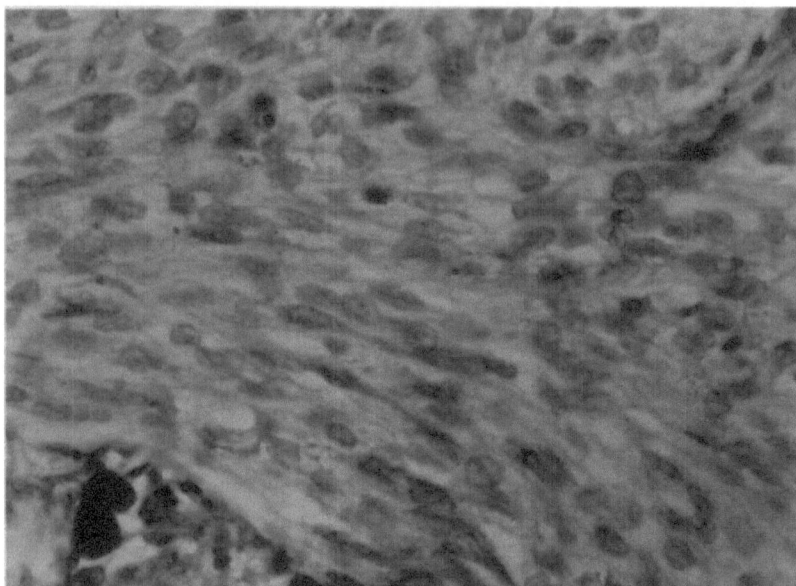

Fig. 35. *Spindle cell tumour*, iris. Thin, elongated nucleus has central chromatin bar (*spindle A*). Slightly plumper cell has elongated nucleus with nucleolus (*spindle B*)

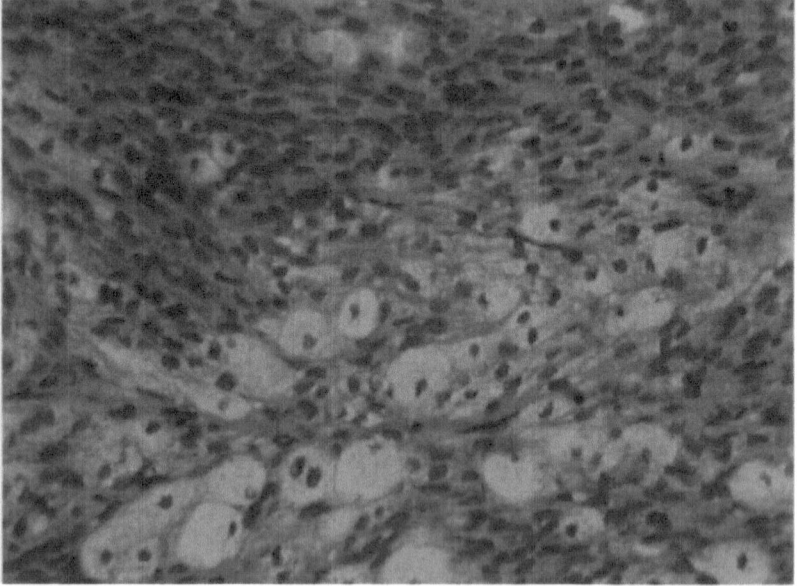

Fig. 36. *Malignant melanoma*, choroid. Balloon cells with lightly pigmented vacuolated cytoplasm

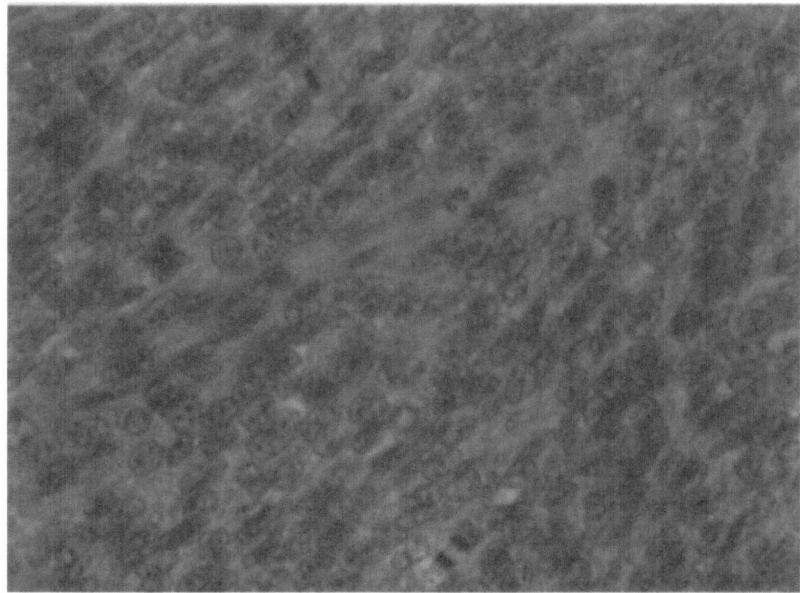

Fig. 37. *Malignant melanoma*, choroid. Spindle B cells are elongated, and the nucleus contains a distinct eosinophilic nucleolus

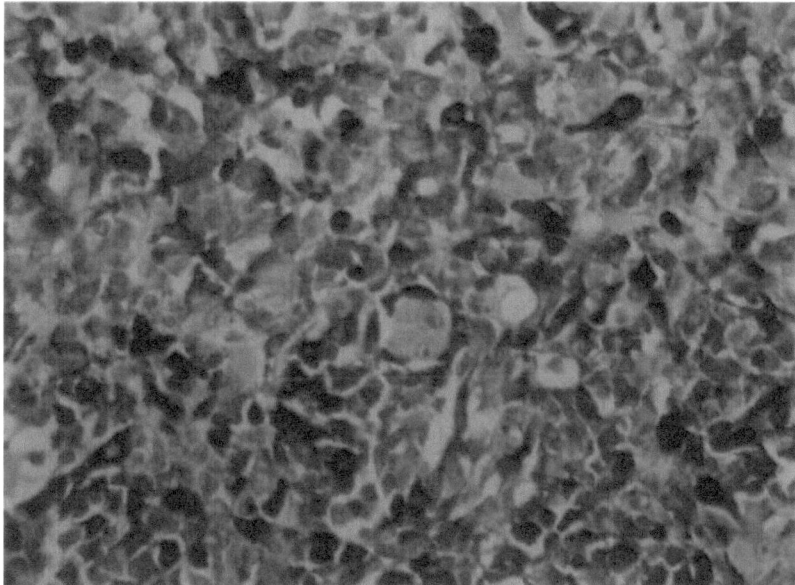

Fig. 38. *Malignant melanoma*, choroid. Epithelioid cells have a rounded nucleus with a prominent nucleolus

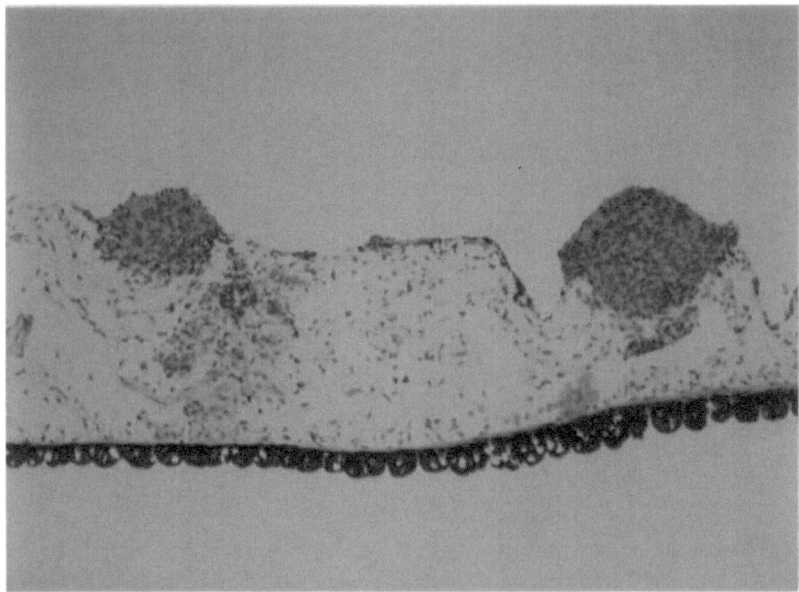

Fig. 39. *Lisch nodules*, iris. Multiple pigmented hamartomatous nodules of iris in a patient with neurofibromatosis

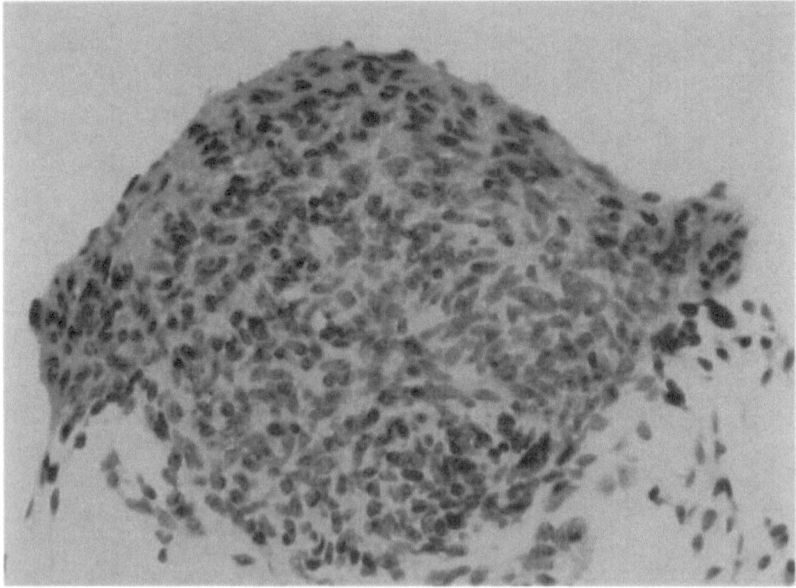

Fig. 40. *Lisch nodule*, iris. Higher magnification of nodule seen in Fig. 39. Focal proliferation of melanocytic cells

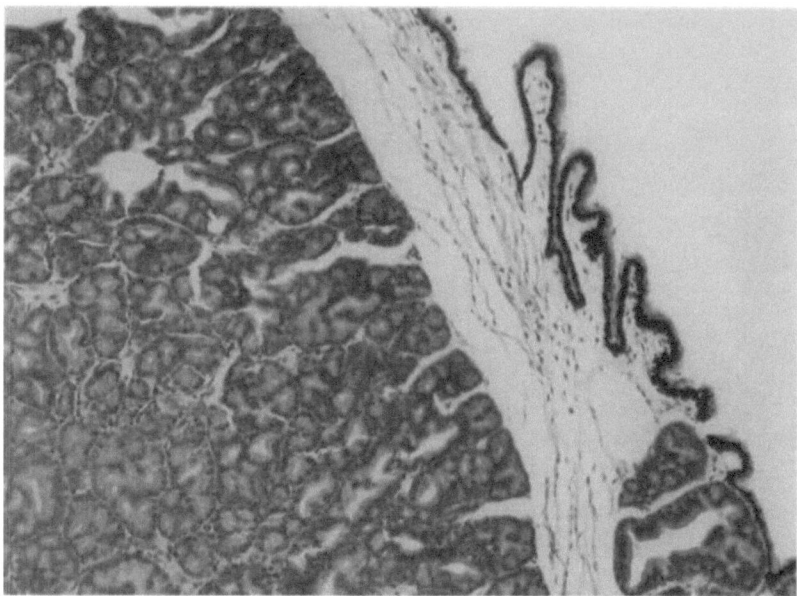

Fig. 41. *Ectopic lacrimal gland tissue*, ciliary body

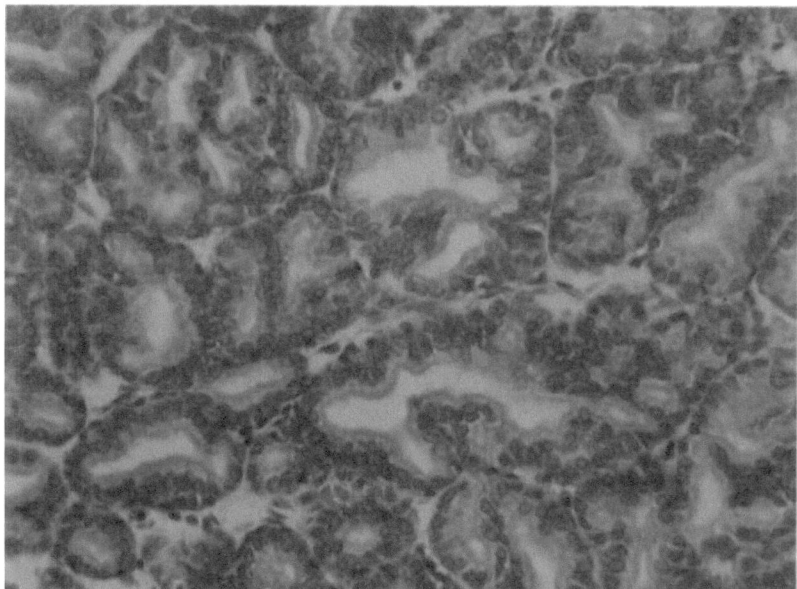

Fig. 42. *Ectopic lacrimal tissue*, ciliary body. Same tumour as in Fig. 41, showing well-formed glands of lacrimal tissue

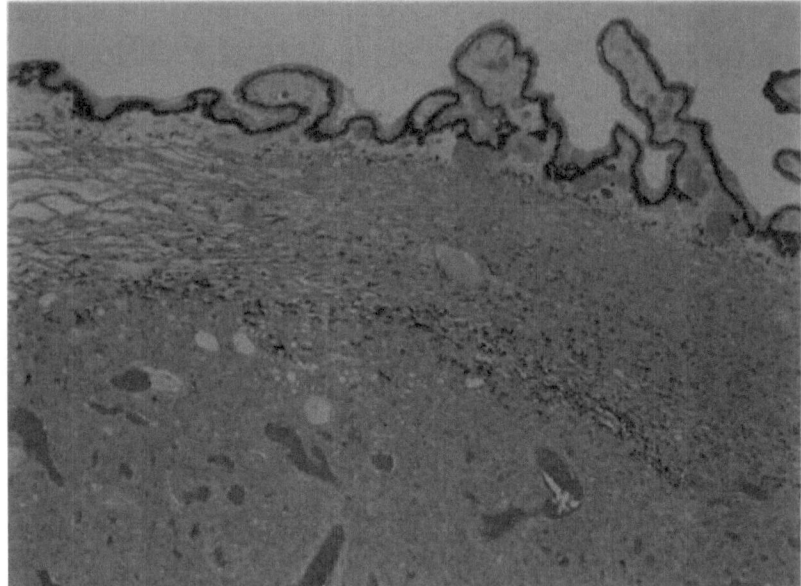

Fig. 43. *Mesectodermal leiomyoma*, ciliary body. Mass confined to ciliary muscle

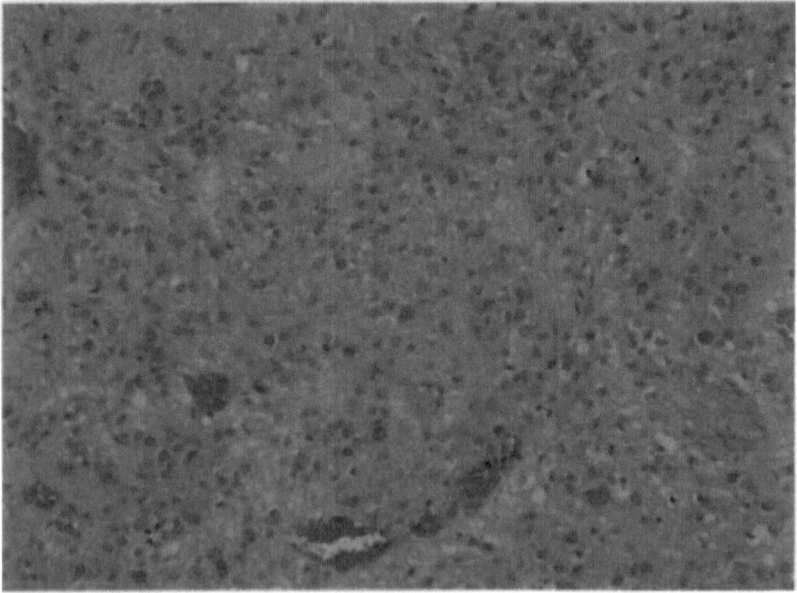

Fig. 44. *Mesectodermal leiomyoma*. Same tumour as in Fig. 43. Interlacing spindle-shaped smooth muscle cells within fibrillar background

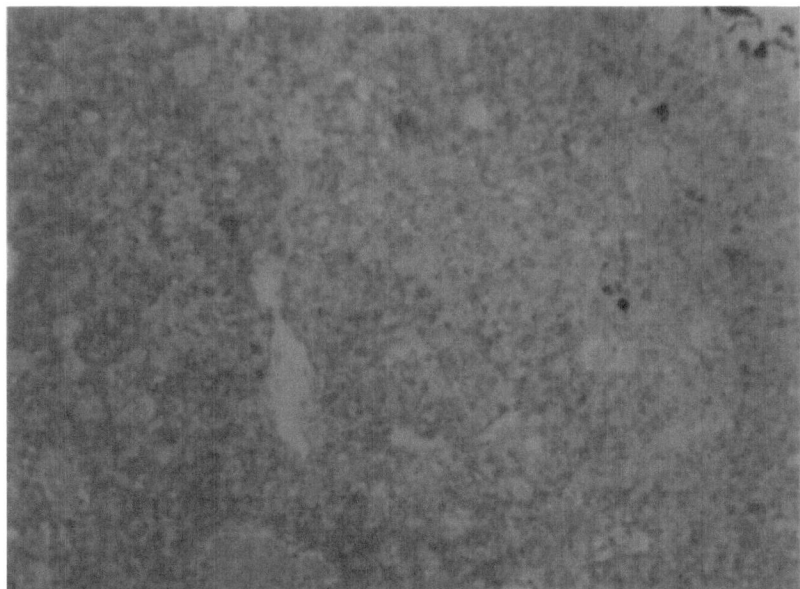

Fig. 45. *Mesectodermal leiomyoma*, ciliary body. Same tumour as in Fig. 43, showing positive immunohistochemical staining for smooth muscle actin

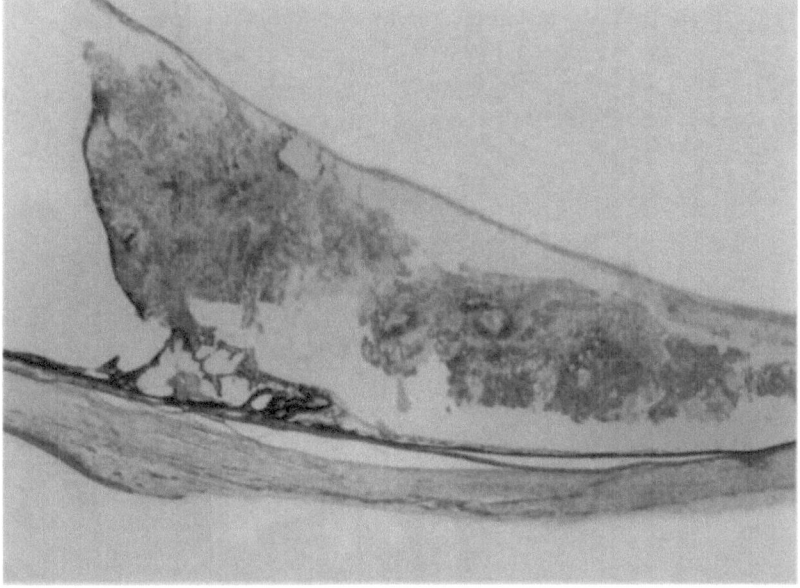

Fig. 46. *Benign, non-teratoid medulloepithelioma*, ciliary body. The ciliary muscle is totally replaced by small, dark tumour cells

74

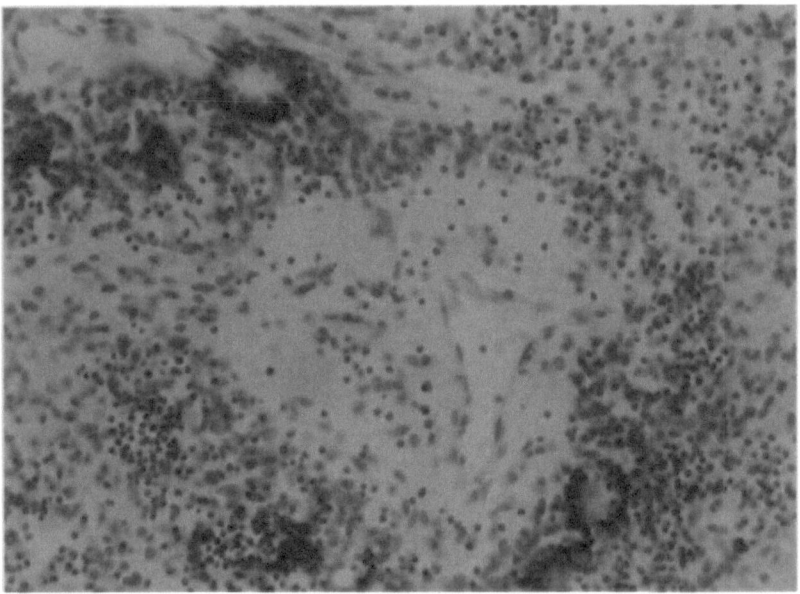

Fig. 47. *Benign, non-teratoid medulloepithelioma*, ciliary body. Same tumour as in Fig. 46. Neuroepithelial cells with rosette formation

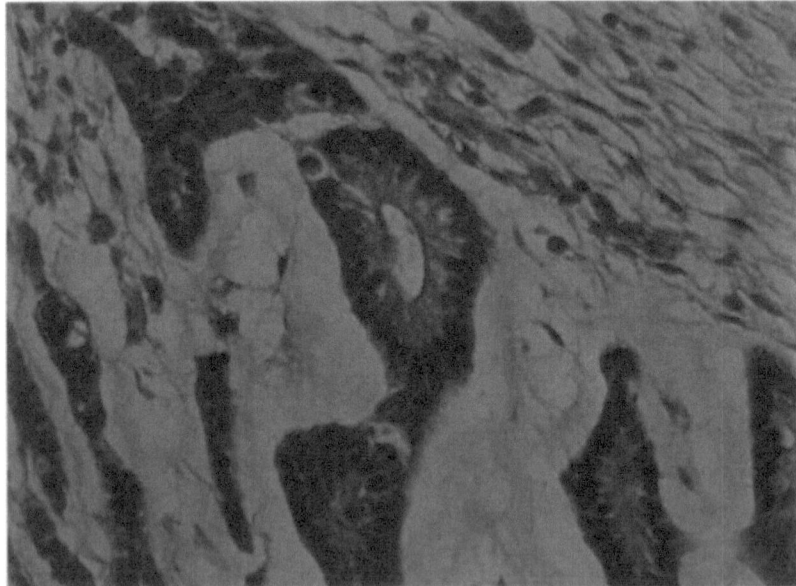

Fig. 48. *Malignant medulloepithelioma*, ciliary body. Multilayered undifferentiated cells akin to those of medullary epithelium

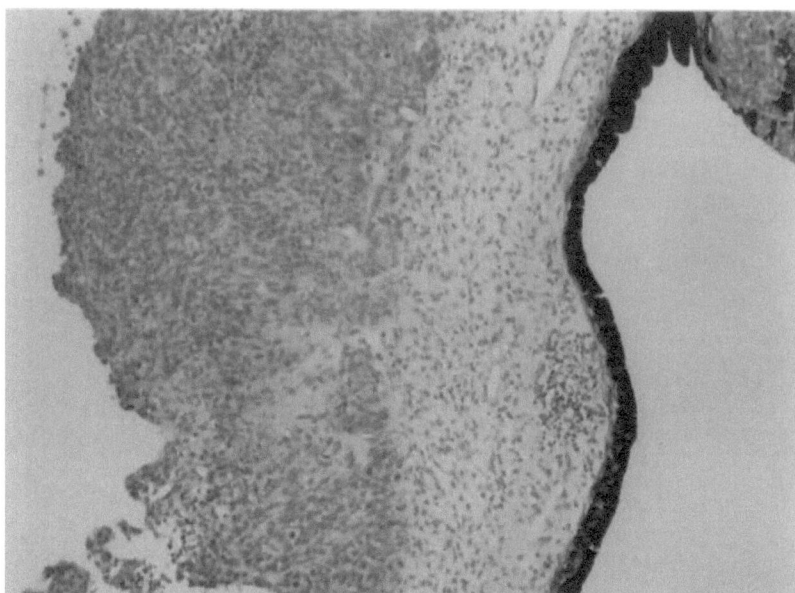

Fig. 49. *Malignant medulloepithelioma, iris.* Tumour extends from the ciliary body to coat the anterior iris surface

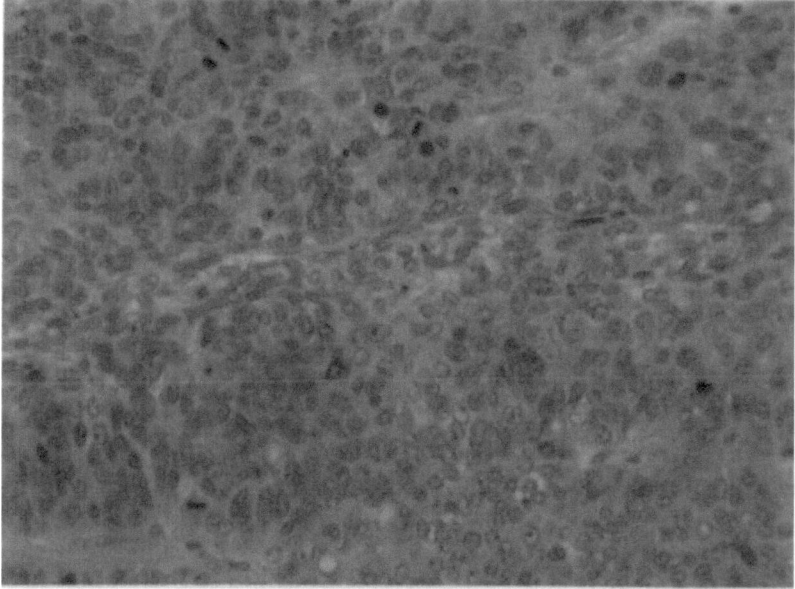

Fig. 50. *Malignant medulloepithelioma*, iris. Same tumour as in Fig. 49. Highly malignant anaplastic tumour. Numerous mitotic figures

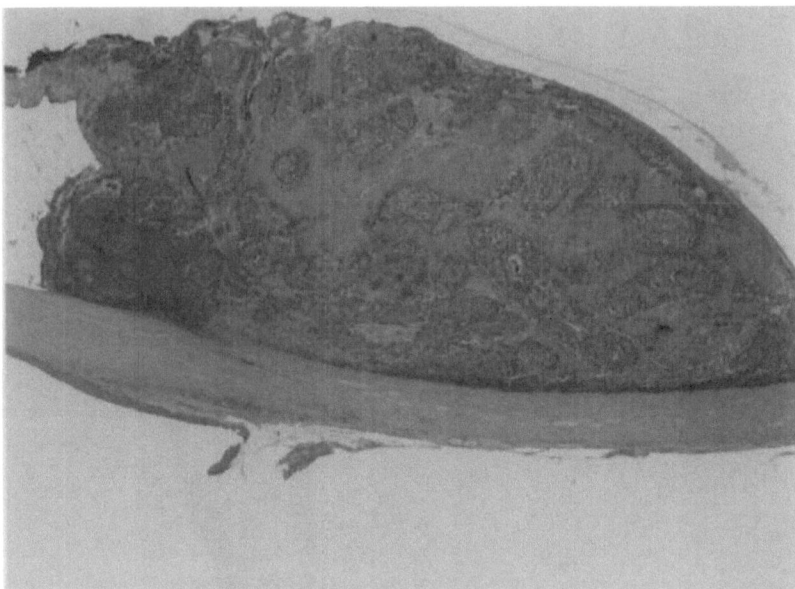

Fig. 51. *Metastasis*, ciliary body. Primary adenocarcinoma of lung, metastatic to the ciliary body and iris. Tumour obscures angle and contains multiple foci of necrosis

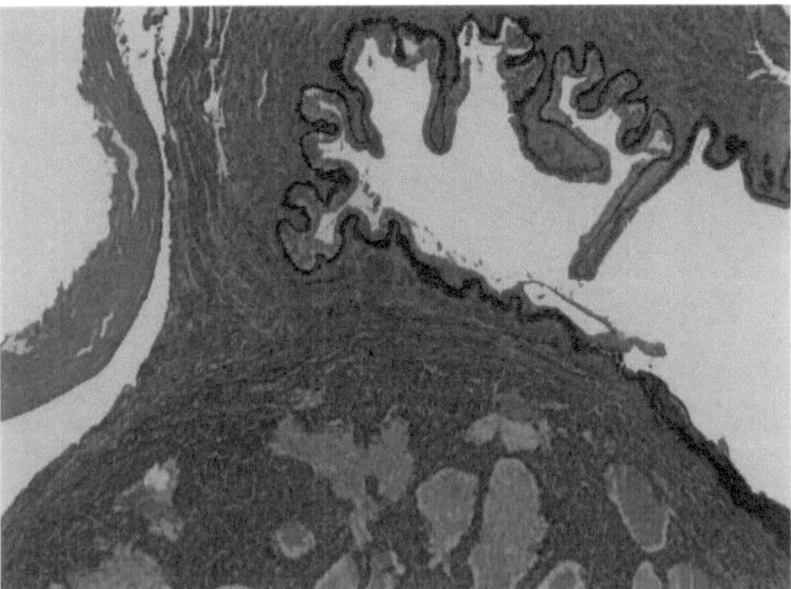

Fig. 52. *Metastasis*, ciliary body. Primary carcinoid tumour of ileum, metastatic to the ciliary body

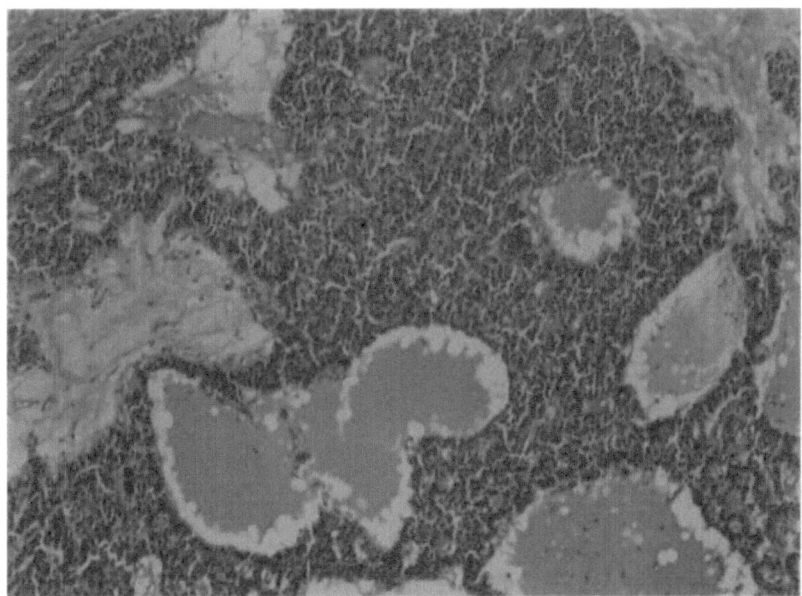

Fig. 53. *Metastasis*, ciliary body. Higher magnification of Fig. 52, showing monoto-
nous pattern of small, dark carcinoid cells

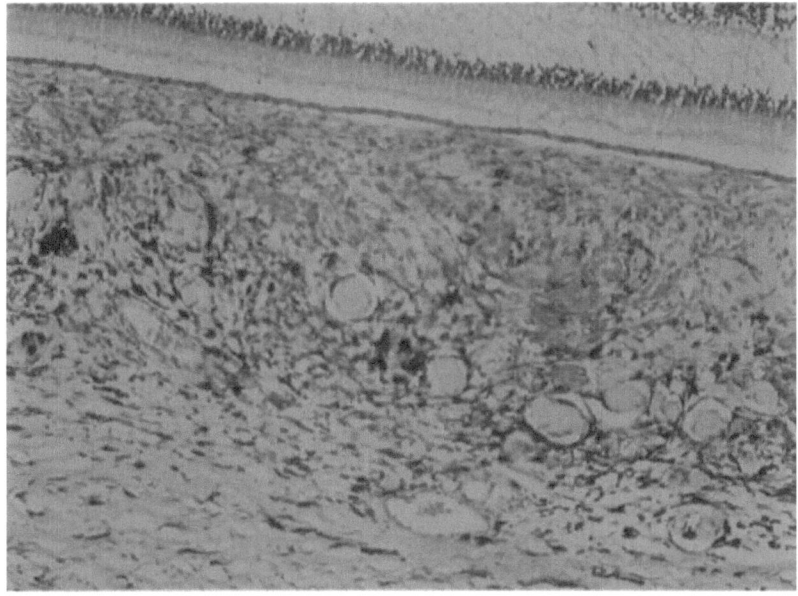

Fig. 54. *Neurofibromatosis*, choroid. Diffuse thickening of choroid by proliferating
Schwann cells and nerve end bulbs

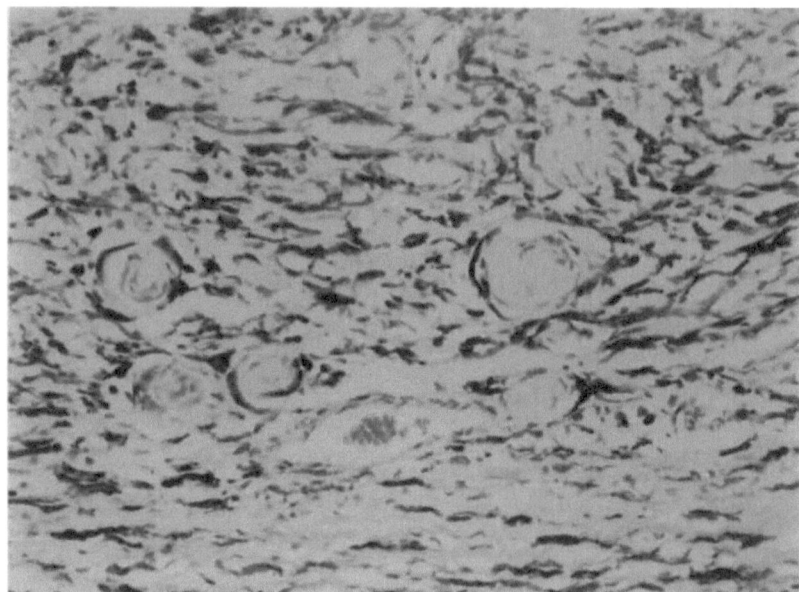

Fig. 55. *Neurofibromatosis*, choroid. Nerve end bulbs appear as rounded configurations surrounded by spindle-shaped nuclei of Schwann cells

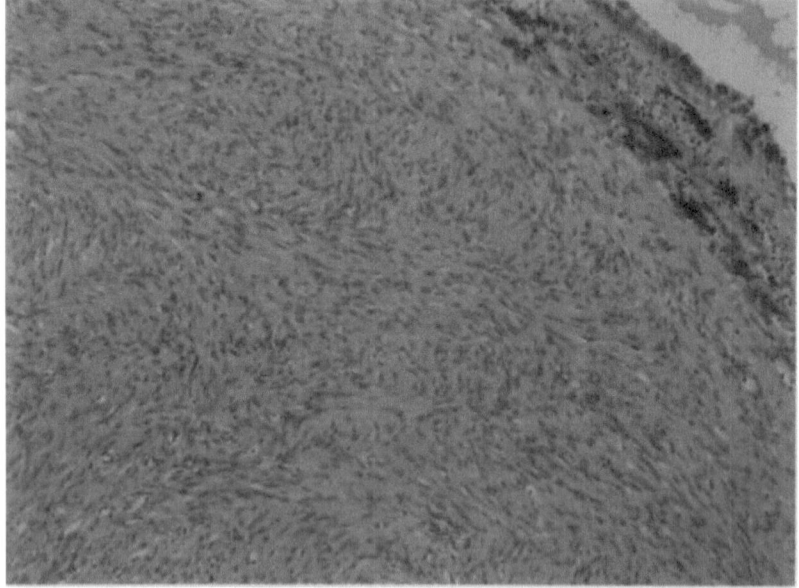

Fig. 56. *Schwannoma*, choroid. Non-pigmented mass occupies choroid

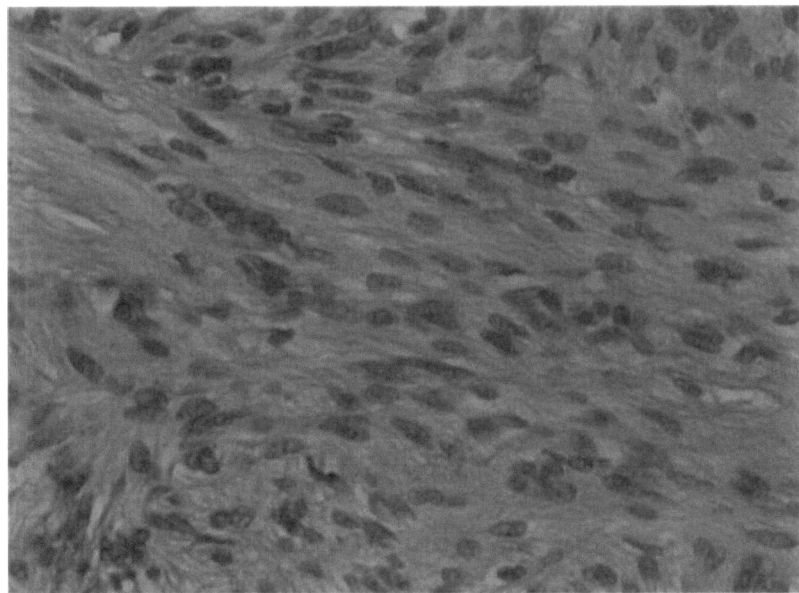

Fig. 57. *Schwannoma*, choroid. Slender, spindle-shaped cells. Nuclei have uniform chromatin pattern

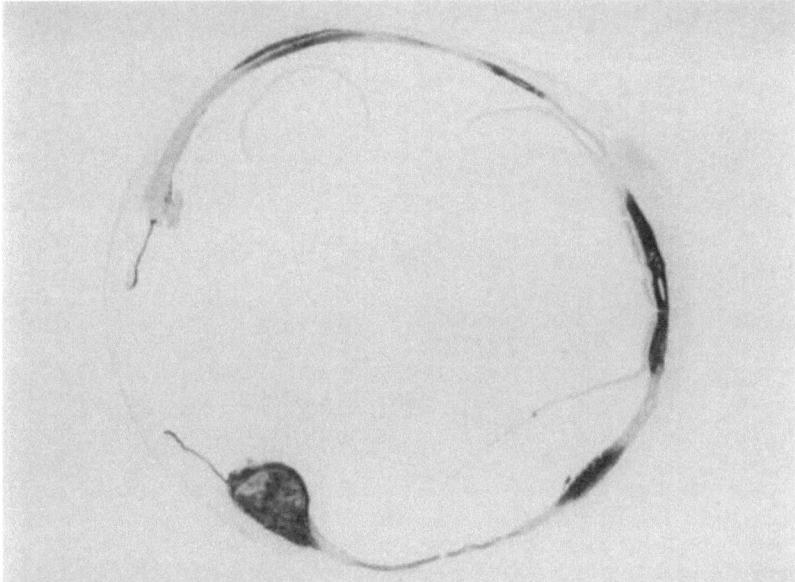

Fig. 58. *Paraneoplastic disease*, uvea. Patient with primary lung carcinoma. Uveal tissue shows diffuse thickening and a ciliary body mass

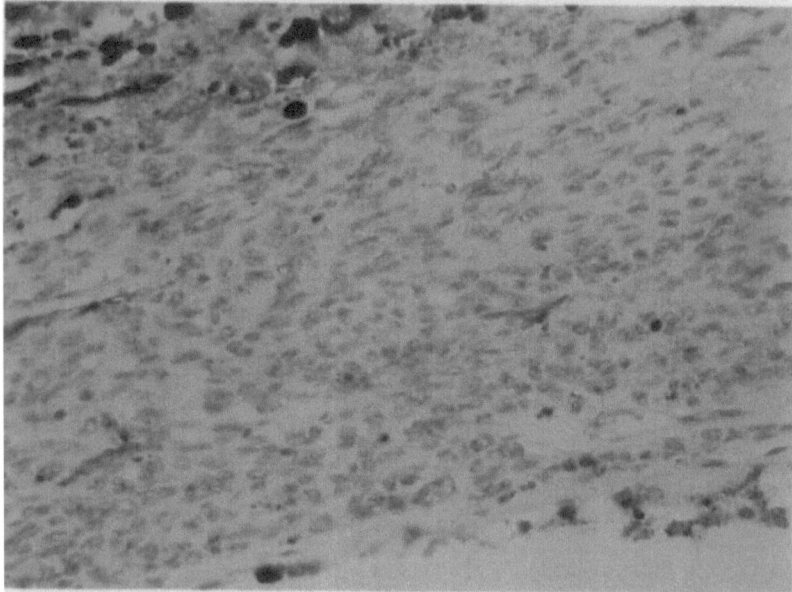

Fig. 59. *Paraneoplastic disease.* Same tissue as in Fig. 58. Proliferating spindle-shaped melanocytic cells within uveal tissue

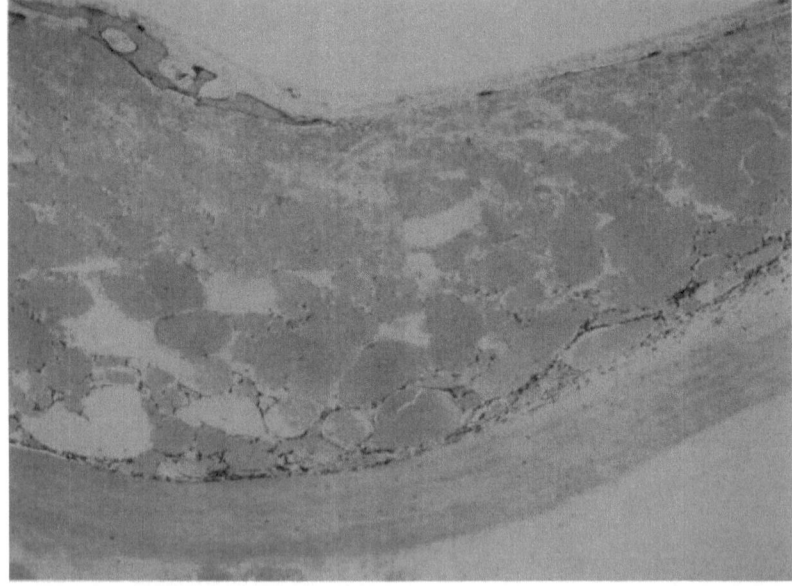

Fig. 60. *Haemangioma*, choroid. Cavernous vascular channels within choroid. Patient with Sturge-Weber syndrome

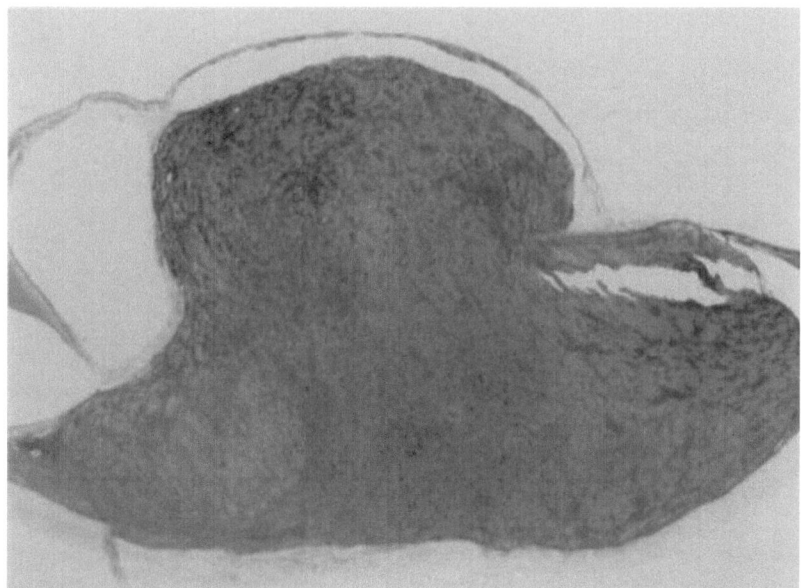

Fig. 61. *Malignant melanoma*, choroid. Mushroom-shaped mass indicating that the tumour has broken through Bruch's membrane

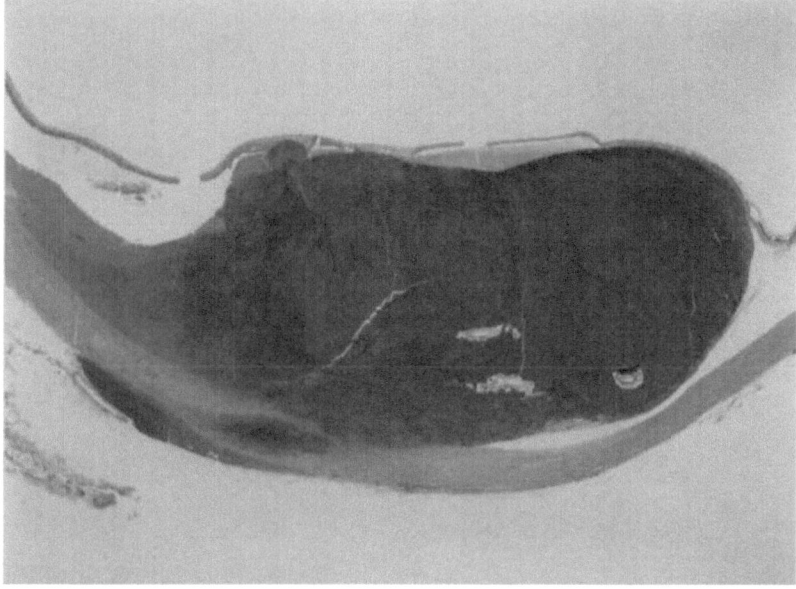

Fig. 62. *Malignant melanoma*, choroid. Tumour extension through sclera via vortex vein

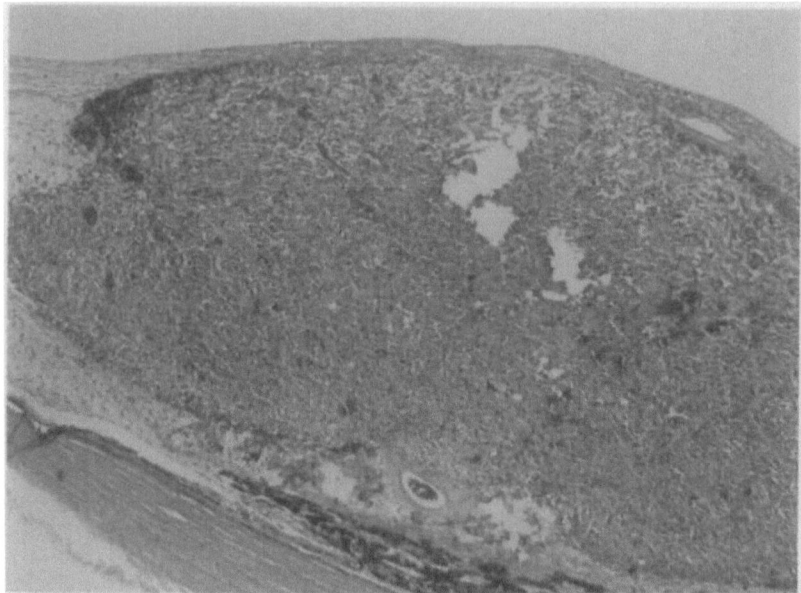

Fig. 63. *Retinocytoma.* Tumour is confined to the retina

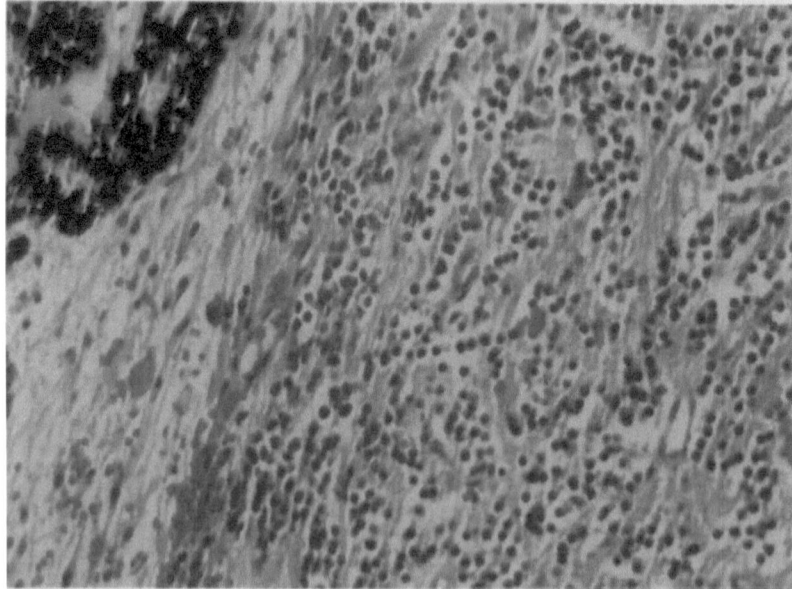

Fig. 64. *Retinocytoma.* Same tumour as in Fig. 63. Small cells with bland nuclei have a small amount of eosinophilic cytoplasm

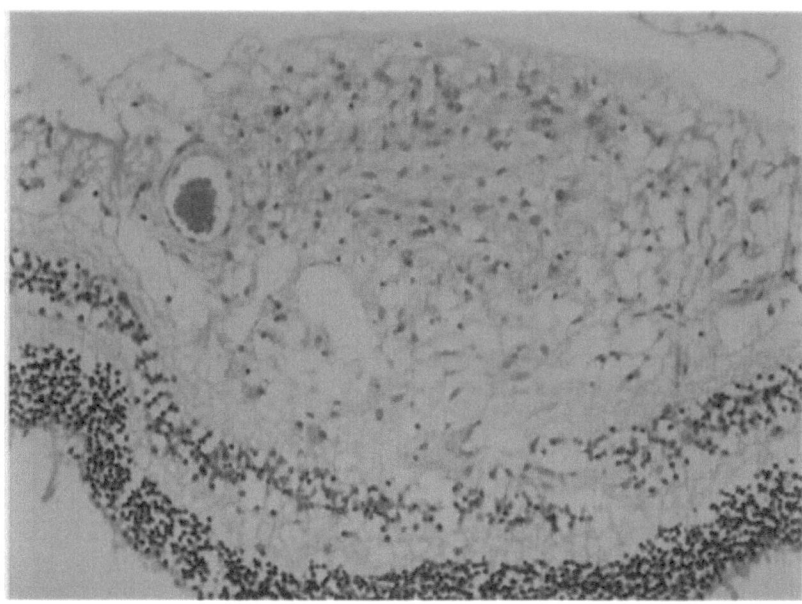

Fig. 65. *Astrocytic hamartoma*, retina. Nodule of spindle-shaped astrocytes within nerve fibre layer of retina. Patient with tuberous sclerosis

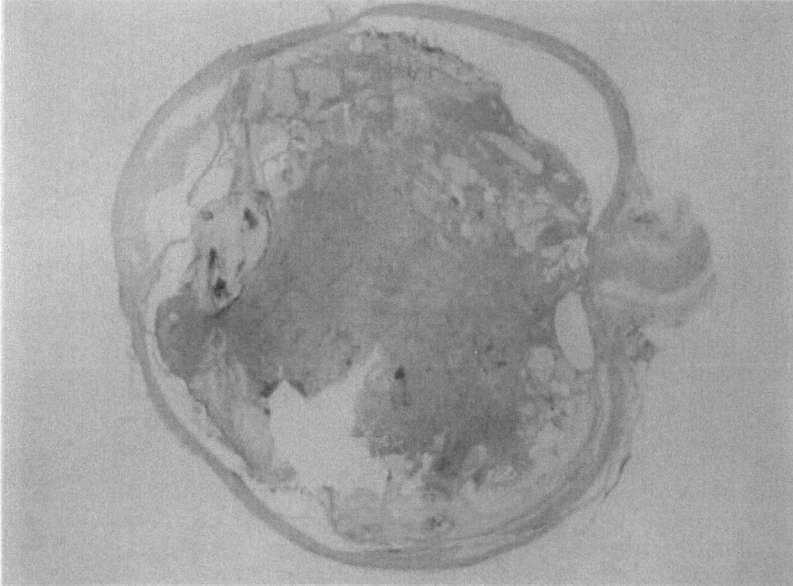

Fig. 66. *Massive retinal gliosis*. The globe is occupied by a mass of proliferating astrocytes

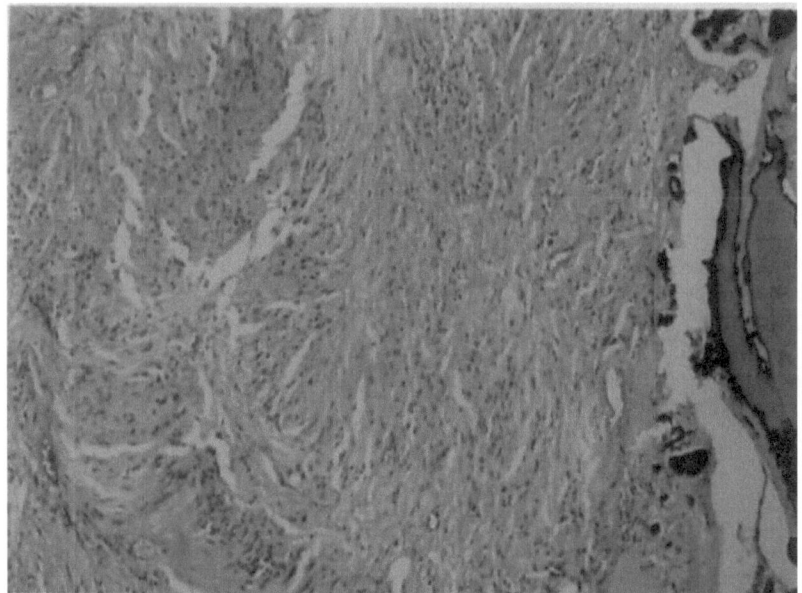

Fig. 67. *Massive retinal gliosis.* Same tissue as in Fig. 66. Interlacing, spindle-shaped astrocytes and focus of bony metaplasia

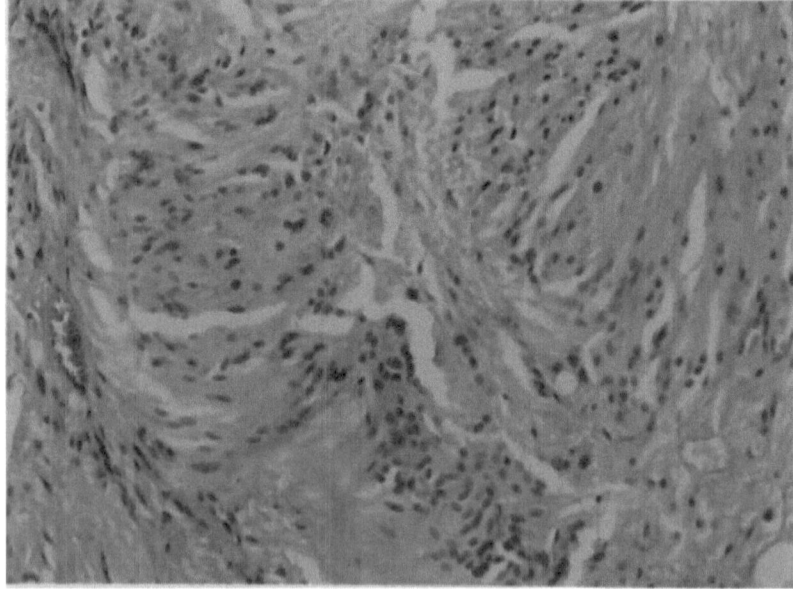

Fig. 68. *Massive retinal gliosis.* Slender, elongated reactive astrocytes

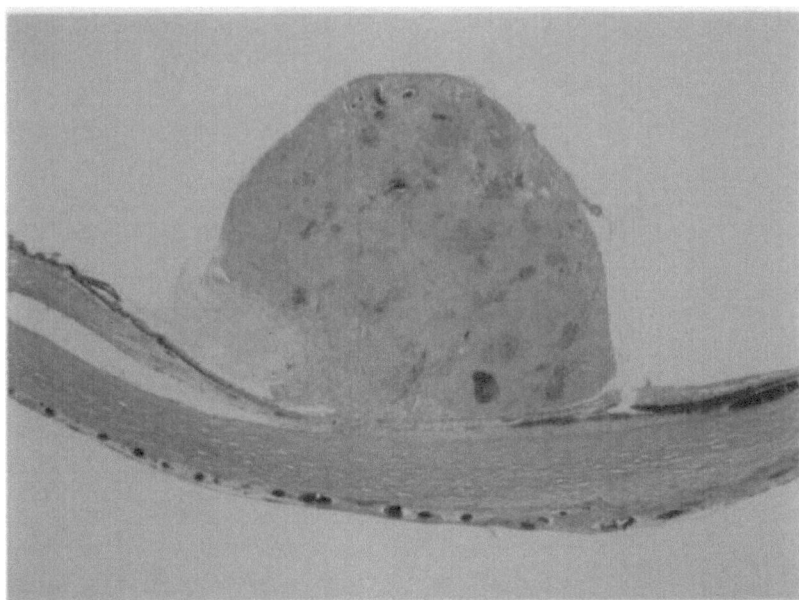

Fig. 69. *Focal reactive gliosis*, retina. Peripheral retina has small focal nodule

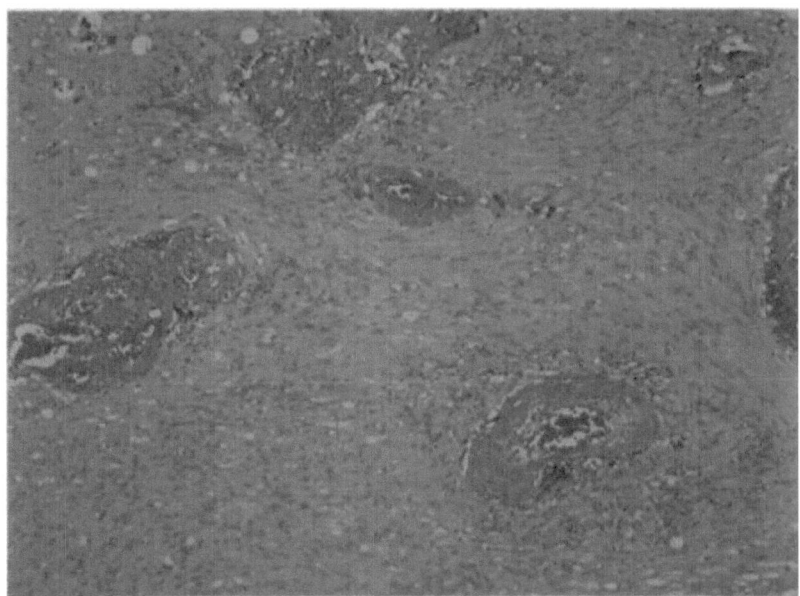

Fig. 70. *Focal reactive gliosis*, retina. Same tissue as in Fig. 69. Thick-walled blood vessels within a background of spindle-shaped glial cells

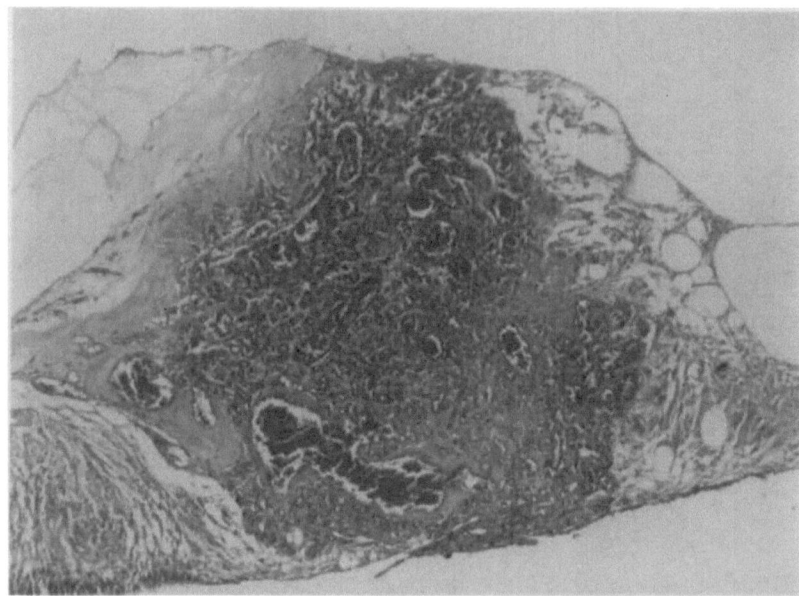

Fig. 71. *Haemangioblastoma*, retina (angiomatosis retinae). Eye from patient with von Hippel disease

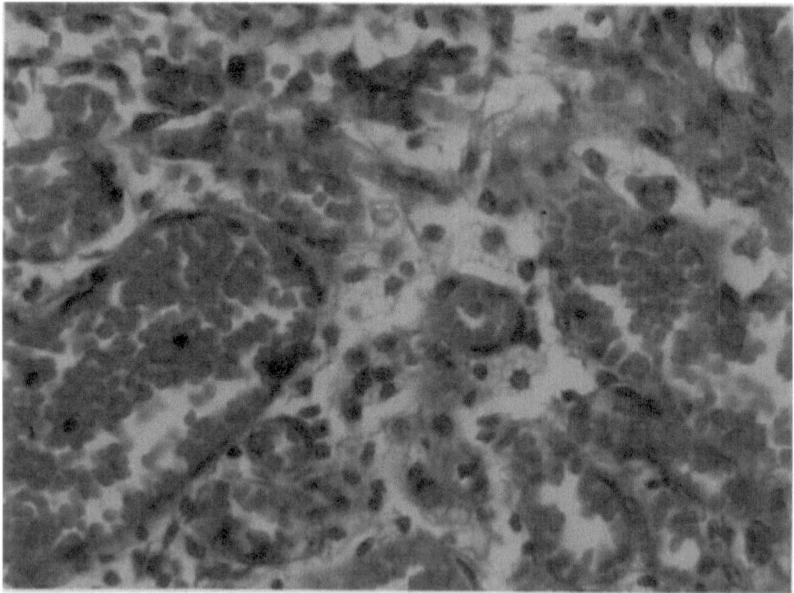

Fig. 72. *Haemangioblastoma*, retina (angiomatosis retinae). Same tumour as in Fig. 71. Thin-walled vascular channels have intervening foamy stromal cells

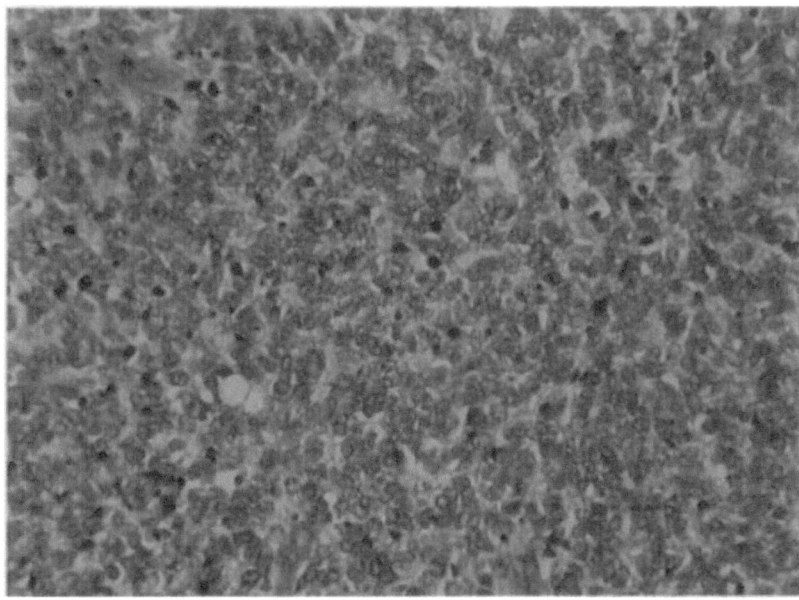

Fig. 73. *Retinoblastoma*, undifferentiated. Sheets of small, dark cells with multiple mitotic figures

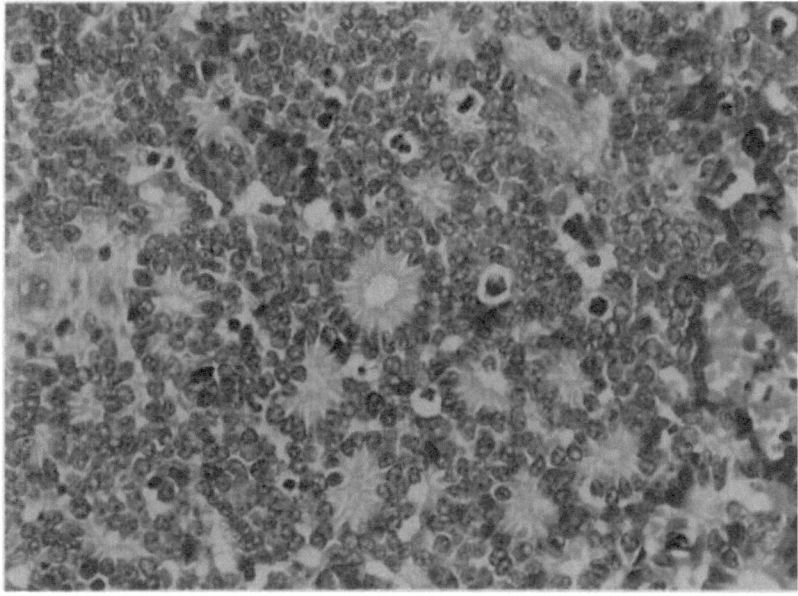

Fig. 74. *Retinoblastoma*, differentiated. Multiple Flexner-Wintersteiner rosettes of uniform size

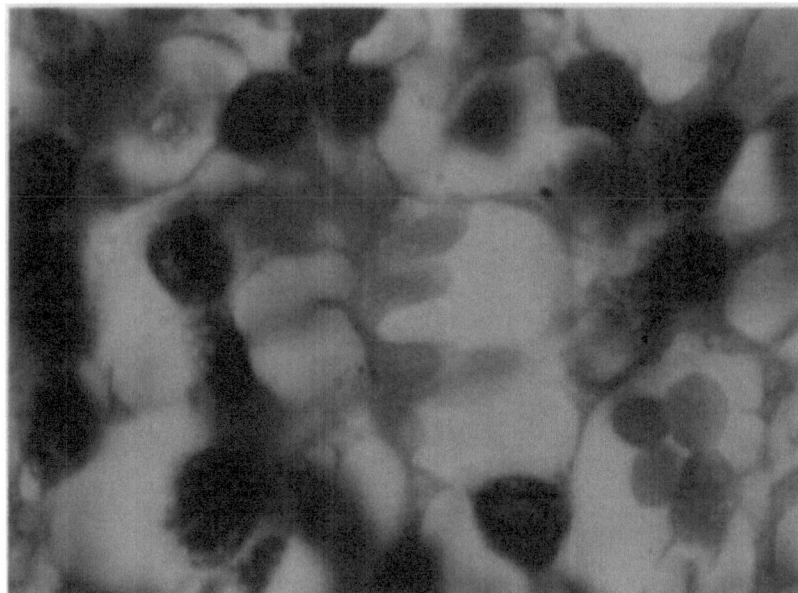

Fig. 75. *Retinoblastoma*, differentiated. Photoreceptor elements in fleur-de-lys arrangement of a fleurette

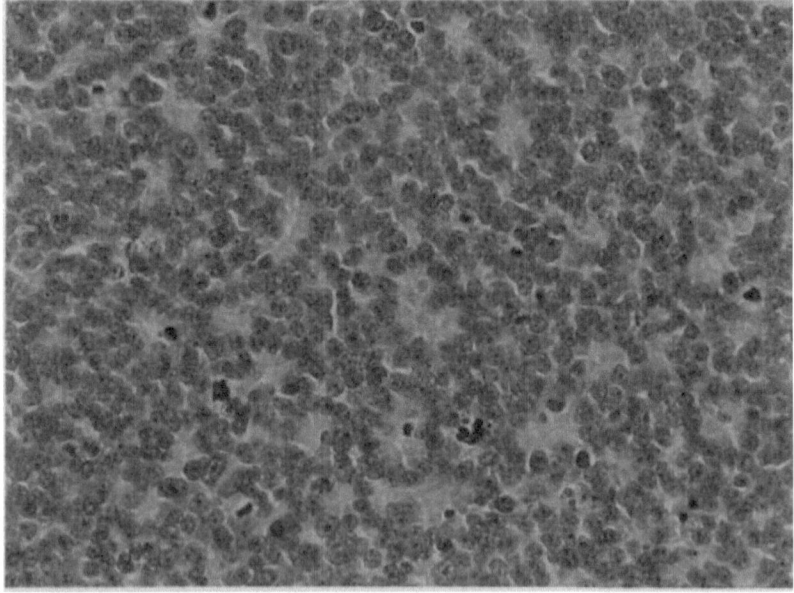

Fig. 76. *Retinoblastoma.* Rosettes of the Homer Wright type of uniform size but lacking in a central lumen

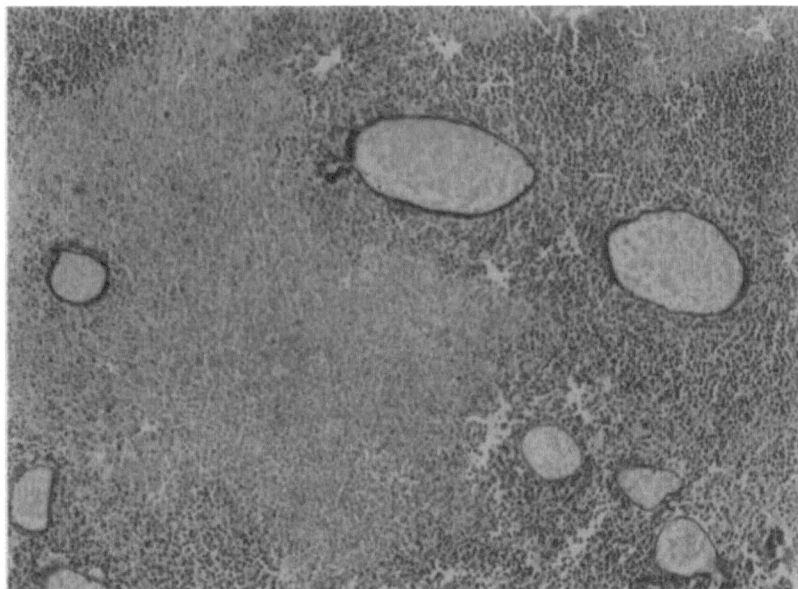

Fig. 77. *Retinoblastoma.* DNA material is deposited in the walls of vessels within a necrotic area of the tumour

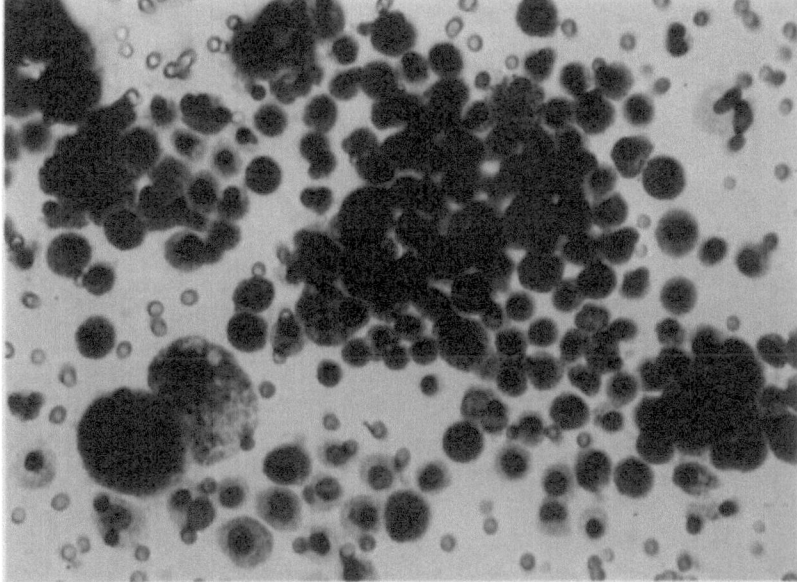

Fig. 78. *Malignant melanoma cells,* vitreous. Metastatic cells from melanoma of skin

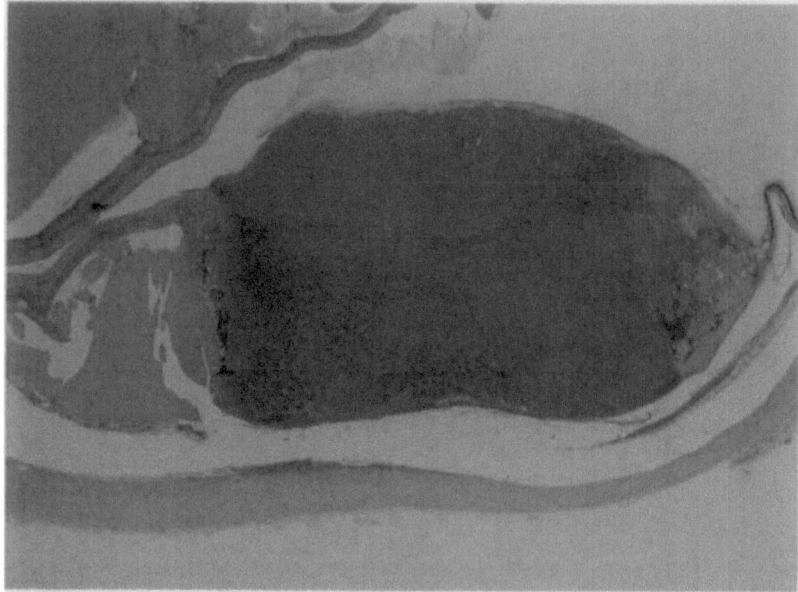

Fig. 79. *Adenoma*, retinal pigment epithelium (RPE). A discrete tumour that is confined to the RPE and has caused secondary detachment of the retina.

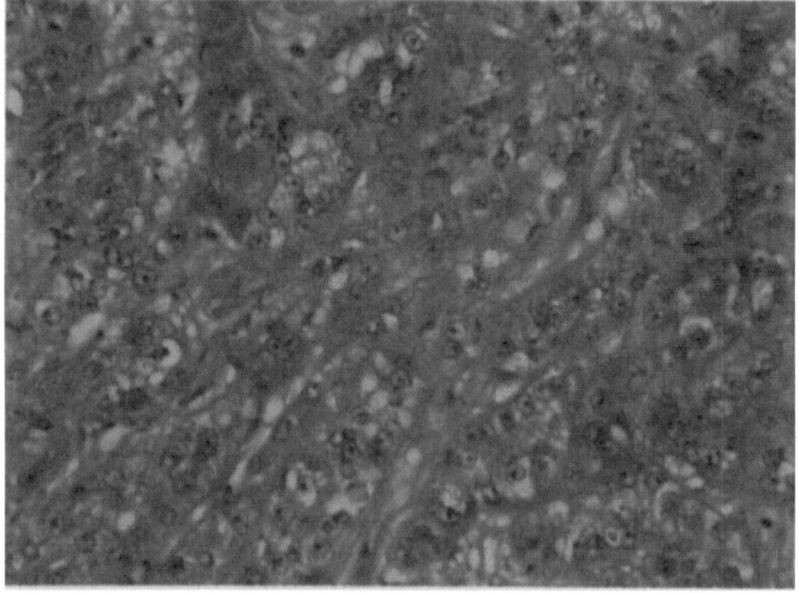

Fig. 80. *Adenoma*, retinal pigment epithelium. Same tumour as in Fig. 79

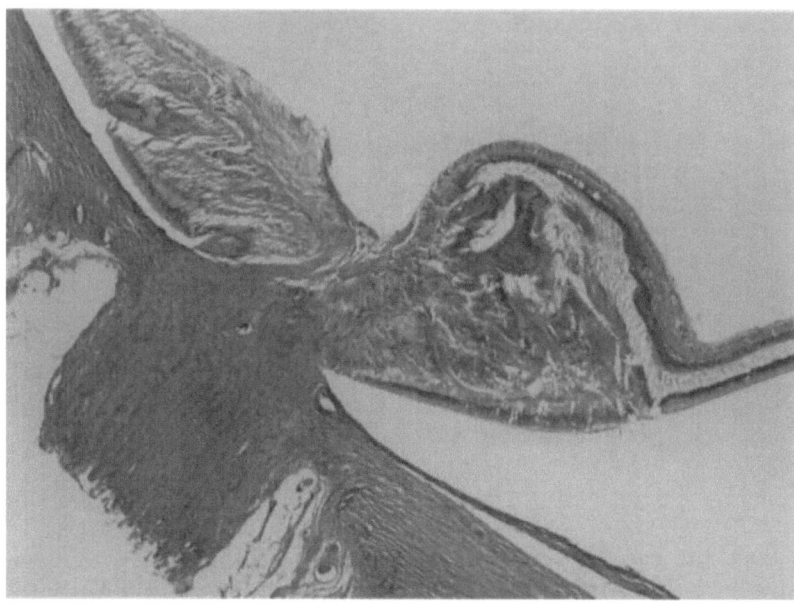

Fig. 81. *Combined hamartoma*, retina and retinal pigment epithelium. Nodule occupies the optic disc, adjacent retinal pigment epithelium and retina

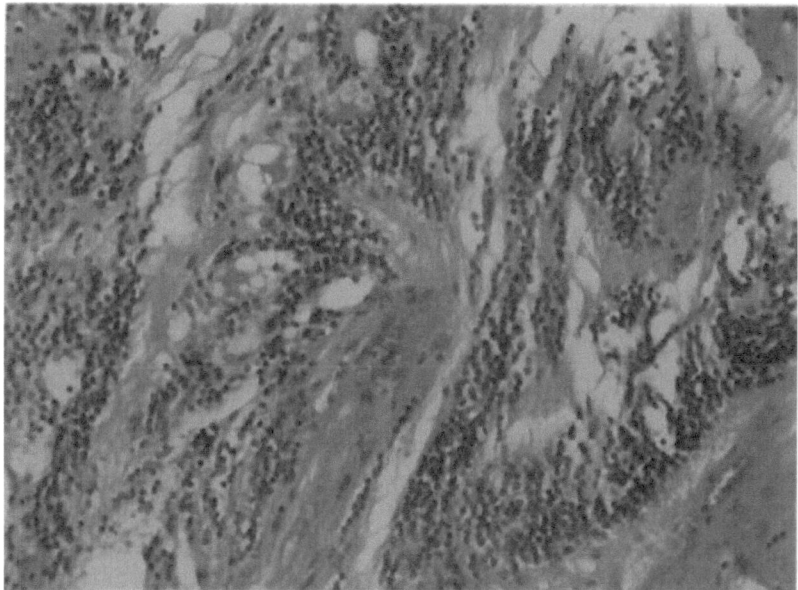

Fig. 82. *Combined hamartoma*, retina and retinal pigment epithelium. Disorganised retinal elements

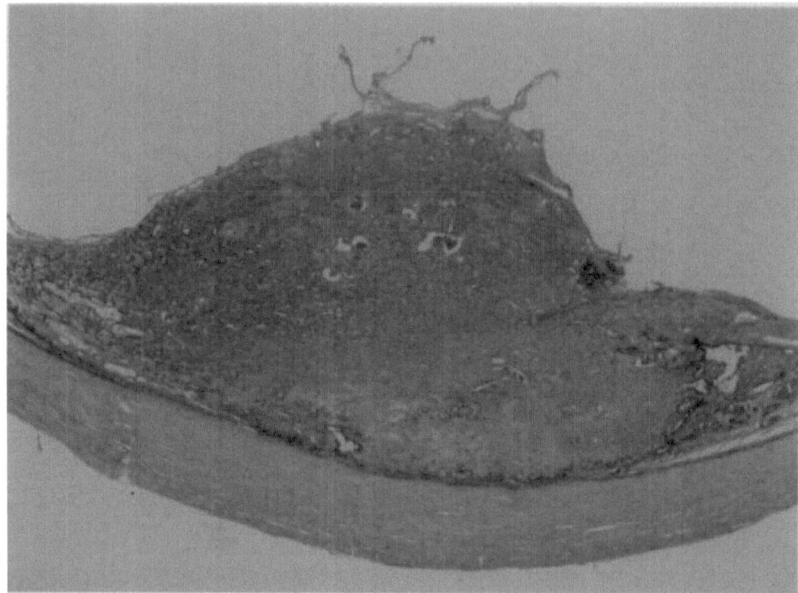

Fig. 83. *Adenocarcinoma*, retinal pigment epithelium. The tumour involves the retina and the choroid.

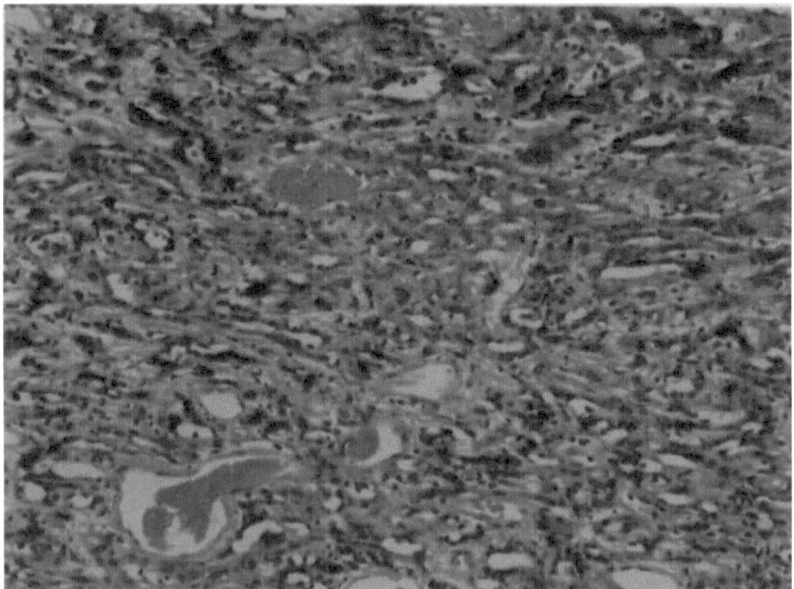

Fig. 84. *Adenocarcinoma*, retinal pigment epithelium. Same tumour as in Fig. 83. Anaplastic cells with pleomorphism and a poor attempt to form glands

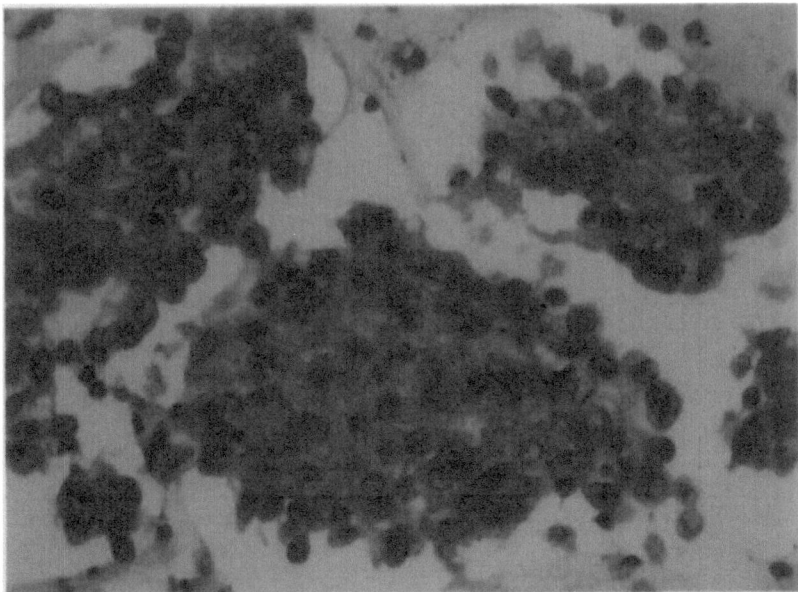

Fig. 85. *Lymphoma*, vitreous. Large cell lymphoma in a vitreous aspirate. The patient also had involvement of the retina and the brain

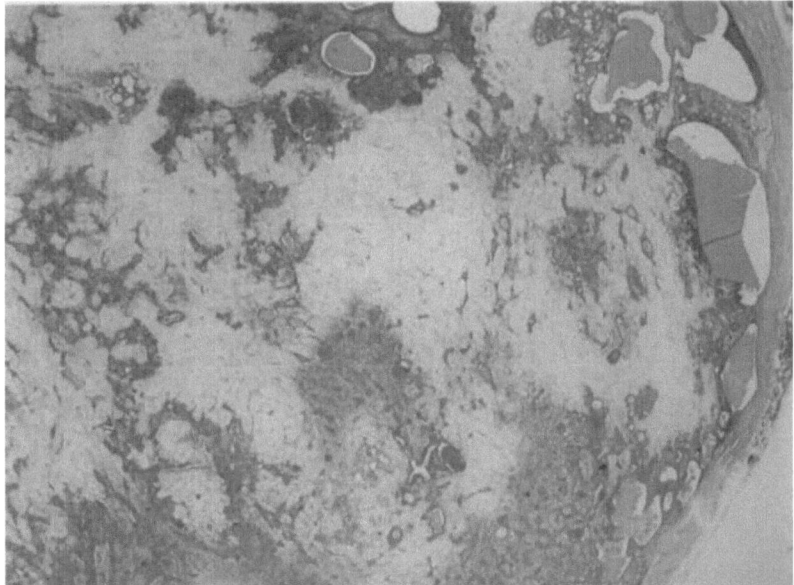

Fig. 86. *Pleomorphic adenoma* (benign mixed tumour), lacrimal gland. Fibrous capsule separates focus of lacrimal tissue from proliferating epithelial and connective tissue components of tumour

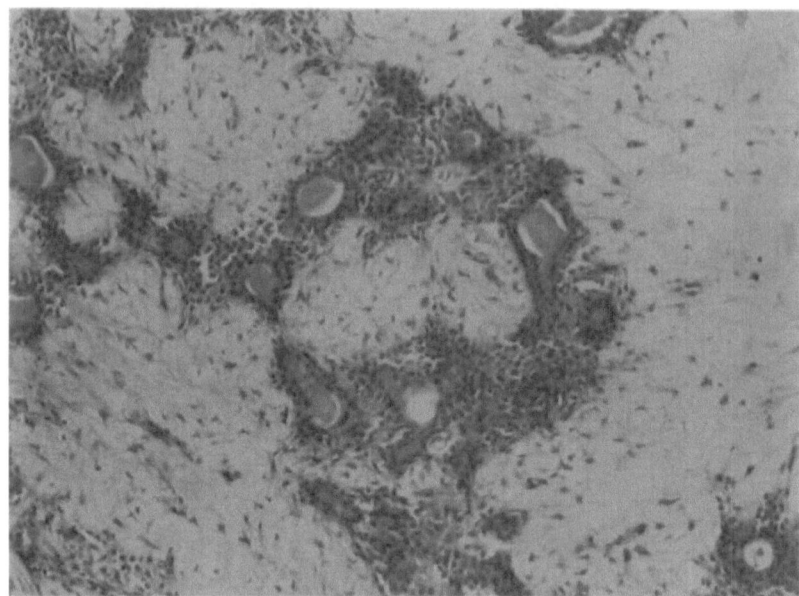

Fig. 87. *Pleomorphic adenoma* (benign mixed tumour), lacrimal gland. Same tumour as in Fig. 86. Ductules with two rows of cells contain eosinophilic secretion. Background stroma is composed of stellate cells

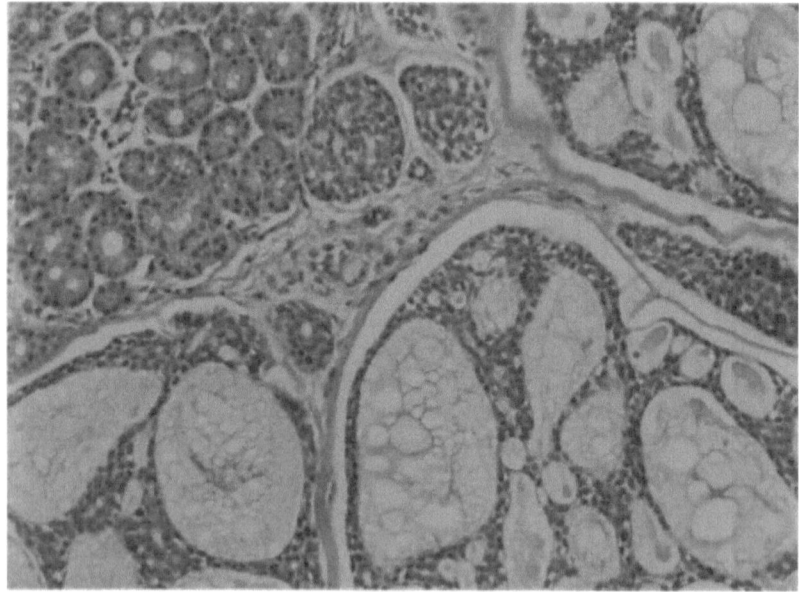

Fig. 88. *Adenoid cystic carcinoma*, lacrimal gland. Swiss cheese pattern

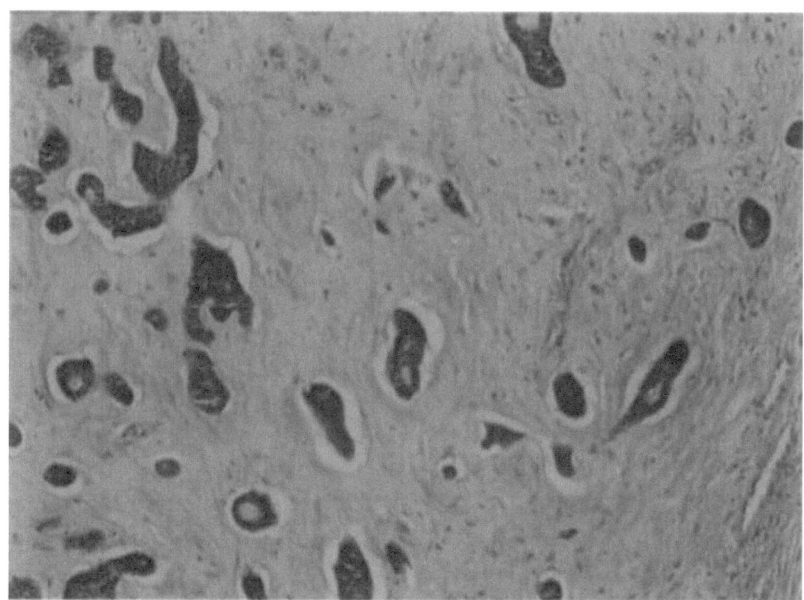

Fig. 89. *Adenoid cystic carcinoma*, lacrimal gland. Sclerosing and tubular pattern

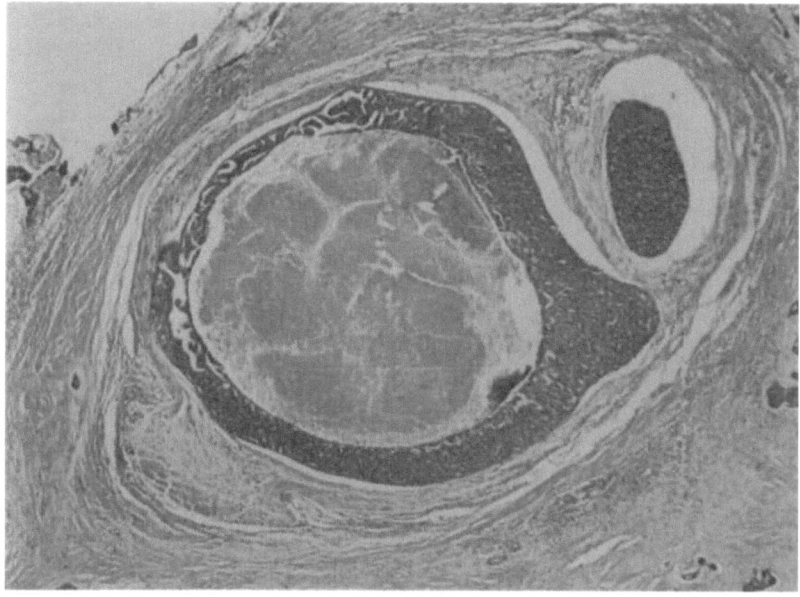

Fig. 90. *Adenoid cystic carcinoma*, lacrimal gland. Comedo pattern

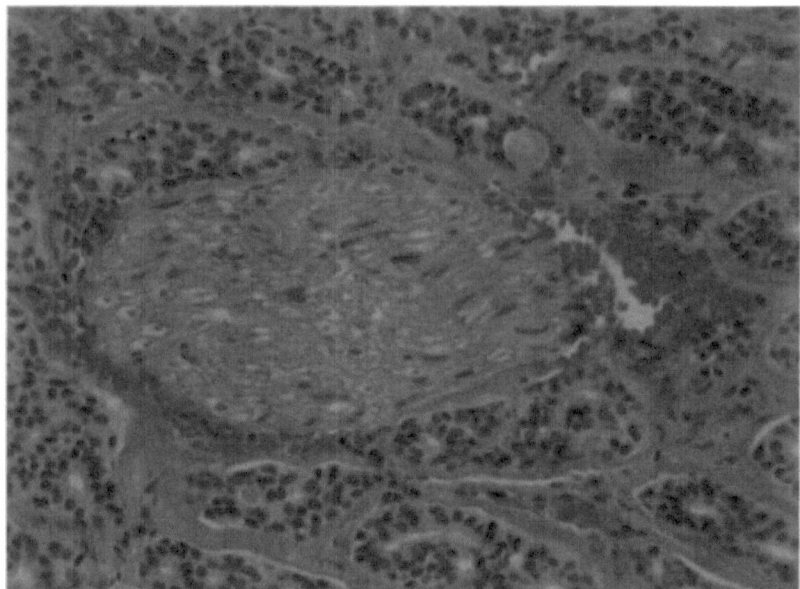

Fig. 91. *Adenoid cystic carcinoma*, lacrimal gland. Perineural invasion

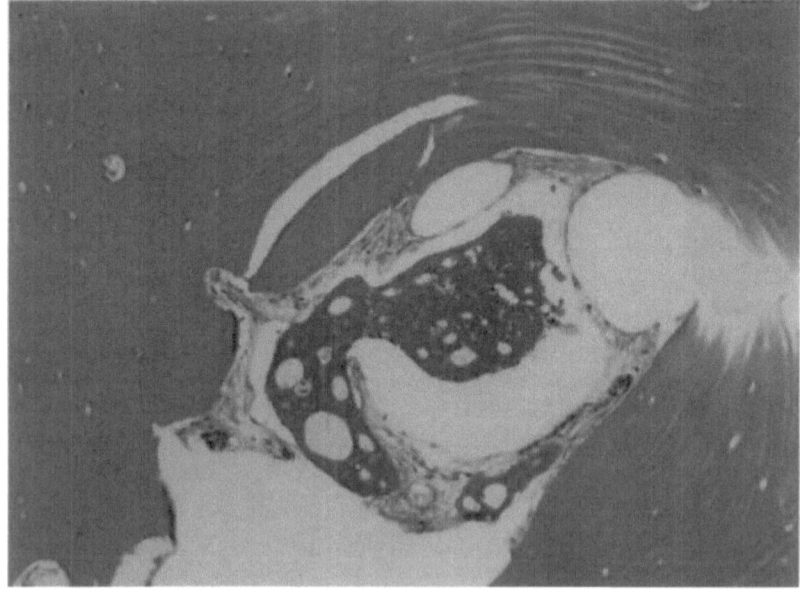

Fig. 92. *Adenoid cystic carcinoma*, lacrimal gland. Invasion of zygomatic bone

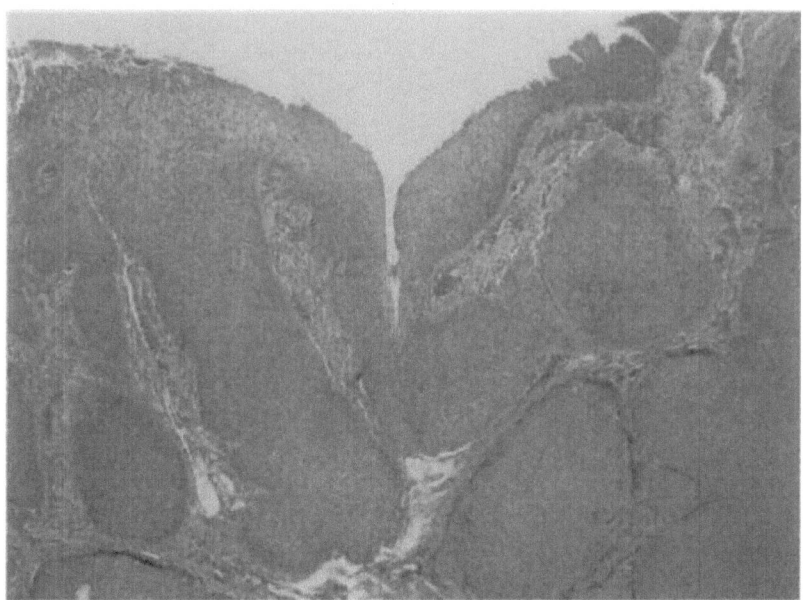

Fig. 93. *Squamous cell carcinoma*, lacrimal duct

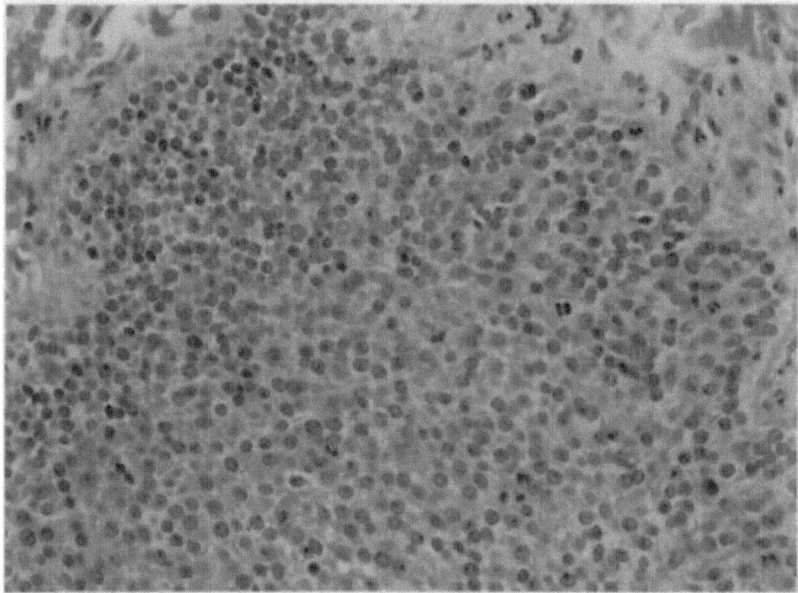

Fig. 94. *Squamous cell carcinoma*, lacrimal duct. Same tumour as in Fig. 93. Infiltrating nests of anaplastic cells

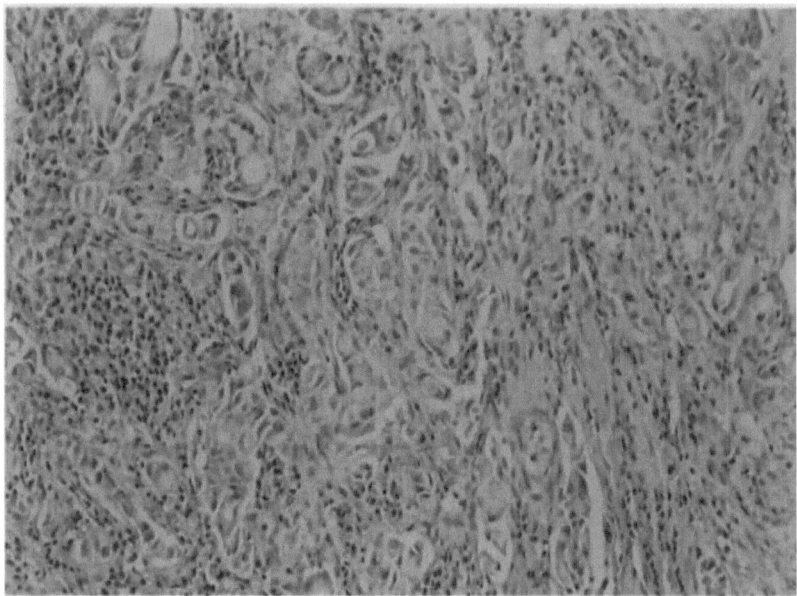

Fig. 95. *Adenocarcinoma*, lacrimal sac. Poorly differentiated mucus-secreting tumour cells

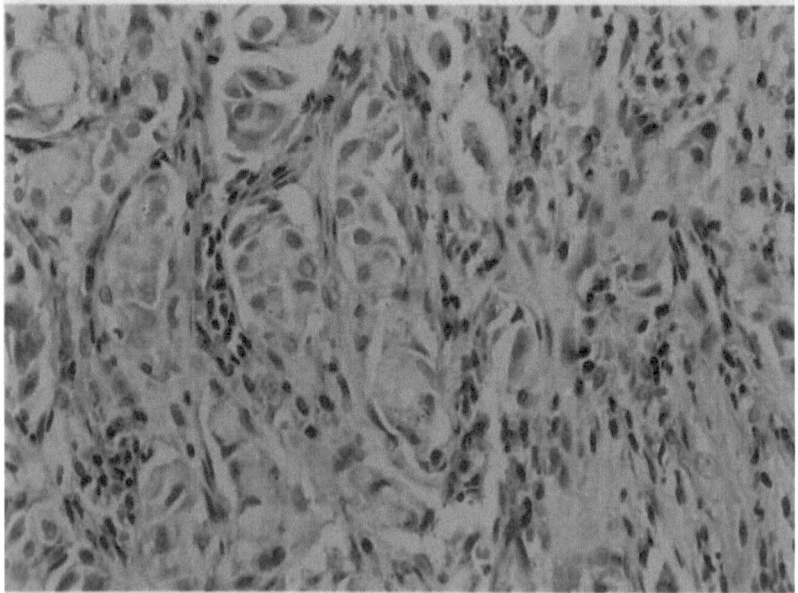

Fig. 96. *Adenocarcinoma*, lacrimal sac. Same tumour as in Fig. 95. Ill-defined glandular pattern of mucus-secreting cells

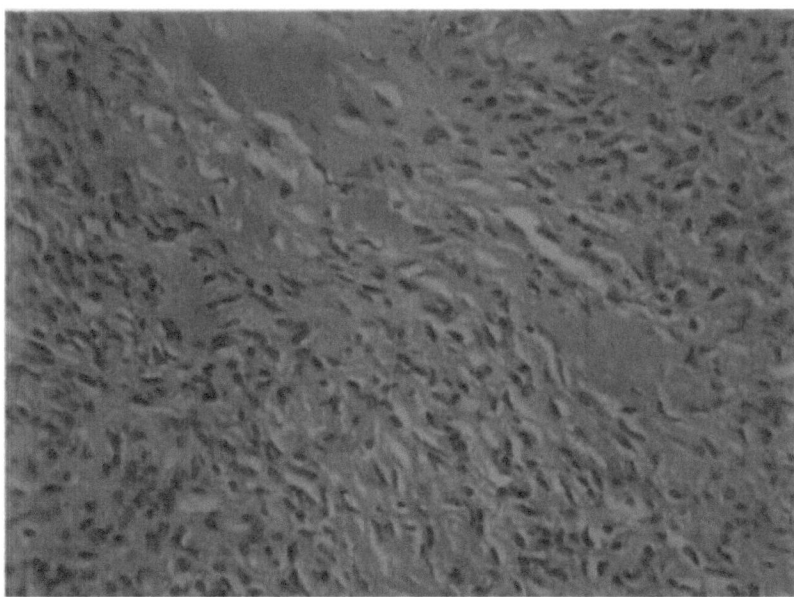

Fig. 97. *Solitary fibrous tumour*, orbit. Interlacing spindle-shaped cells and inter-weaving collagen fibres are a characteristic feature of the tumour

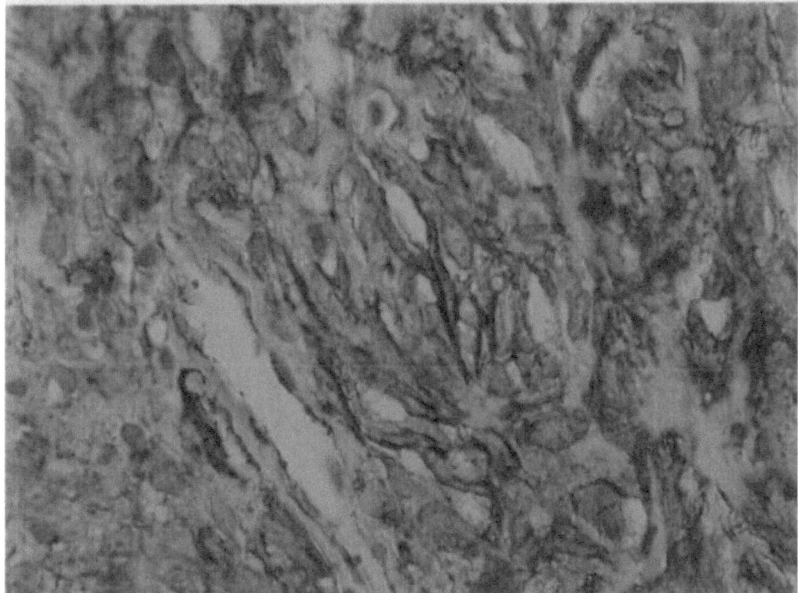

Fig. 98. *Solitary fibrous tumour*, orbit. Same tumour as in Fig. 97. Positive staining with CD34

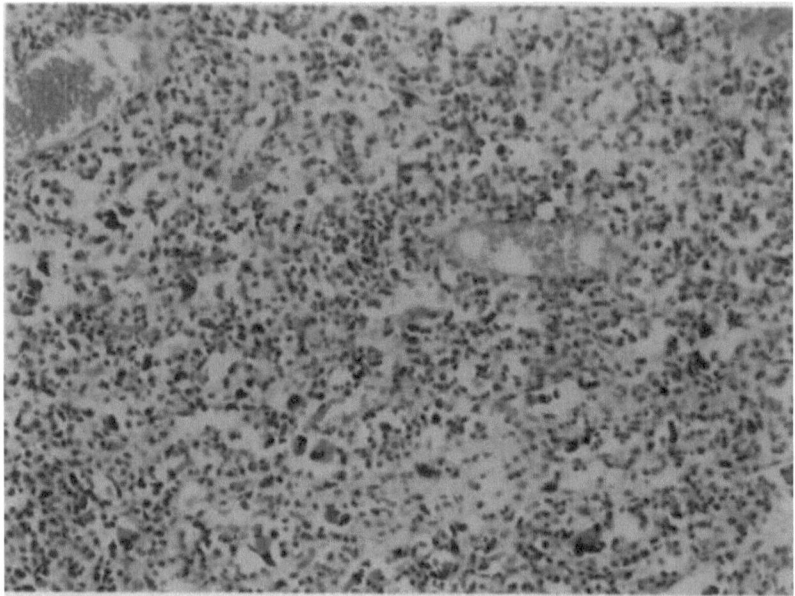

Fig. 99. *Embryonal rhabdomyosarcoma*, orbit. Admixture of small, dark round cells and spindle-shaped cells

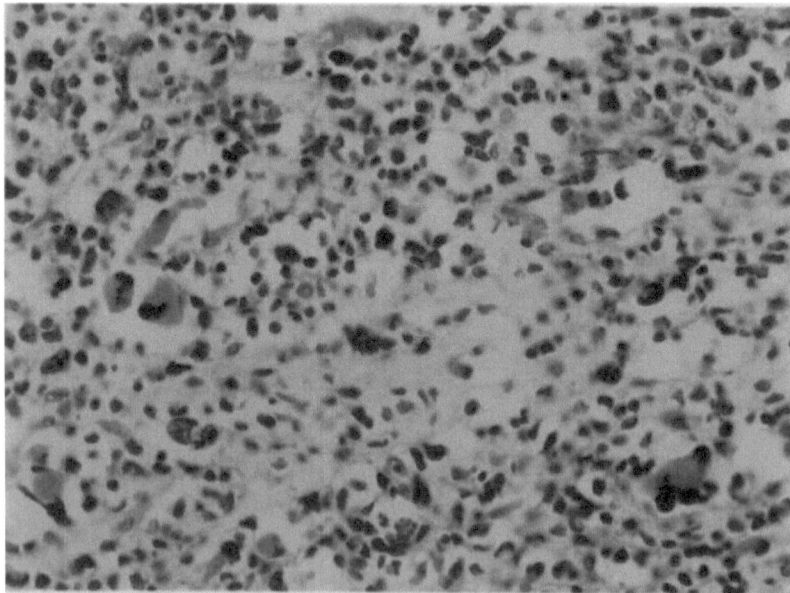

Fig. 100. *Embryonal rhabdomyosarcoma*, orbit. Same tumour as in Fig. 99. Primitive rhabdomyoblasts appear as irregular polygonal cells with deep eosinophilic cytoplasm

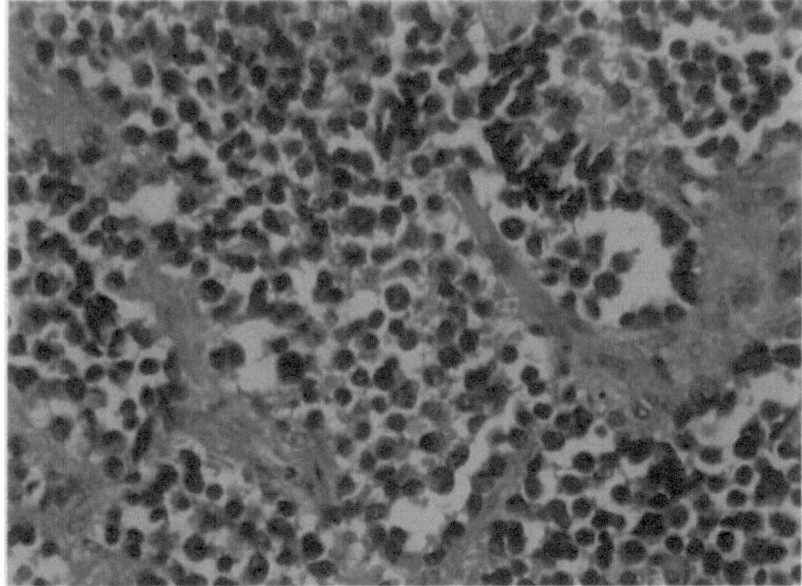

Fig. 101. *Alveolar rhabdomyosarcoma*, orbit. Fibrous stromal septa lined by, and containing, poorly differentiated tumour cells

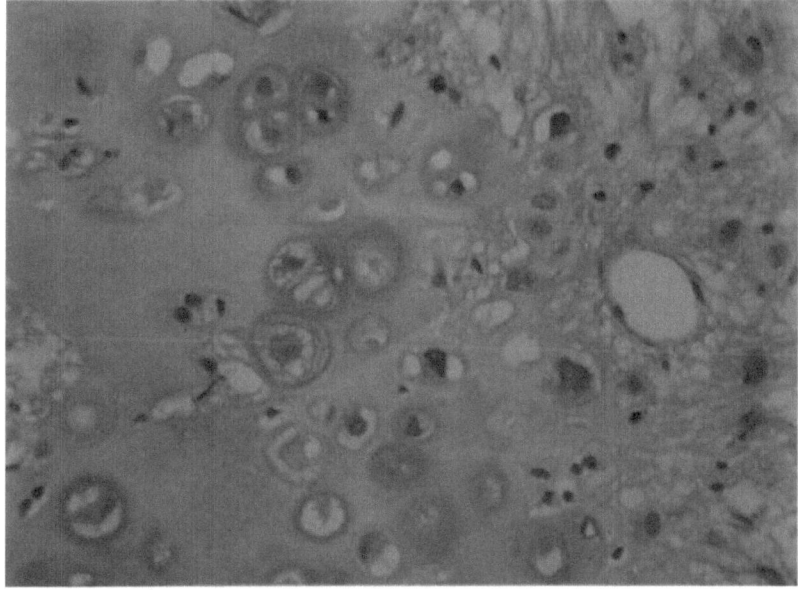

Fig. 102. *Chondrosarcoma*, orbit. Large chondrocytes lie within lacunae

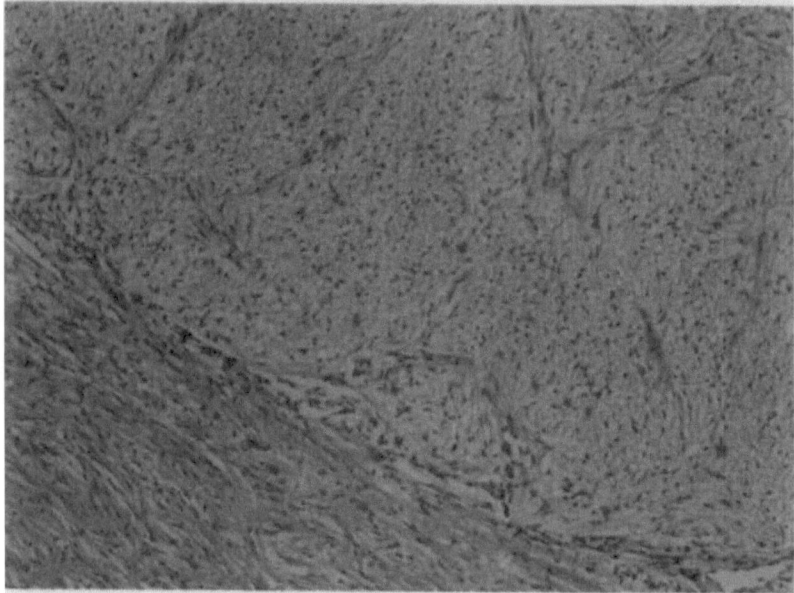

Fig. 103. *Astrocytoma*, optic nerve. Increased cellularity of nerve and thickened meninges

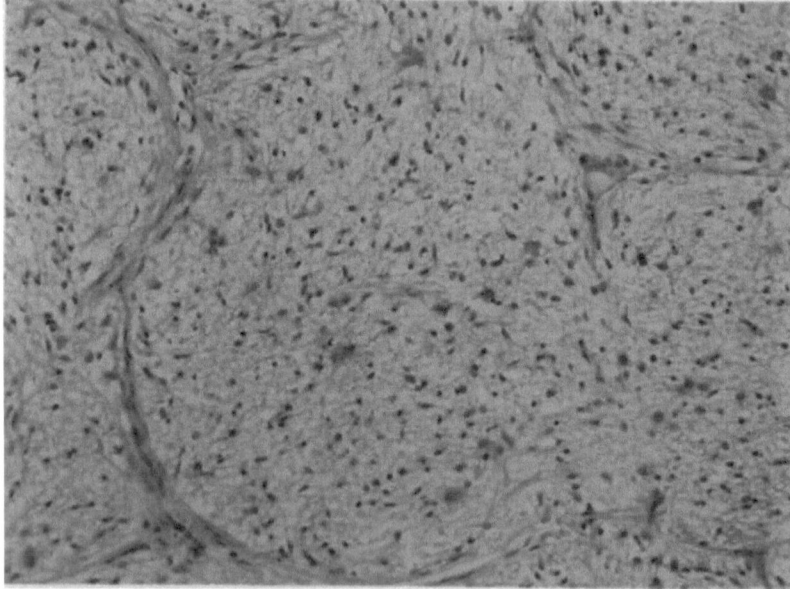

Fig. 104. *Astrocytoma*, optic nerve. Grade 2 glioma. Increased cellularity of nerve. Astrocytes are enlarged and have visible cytoplasm

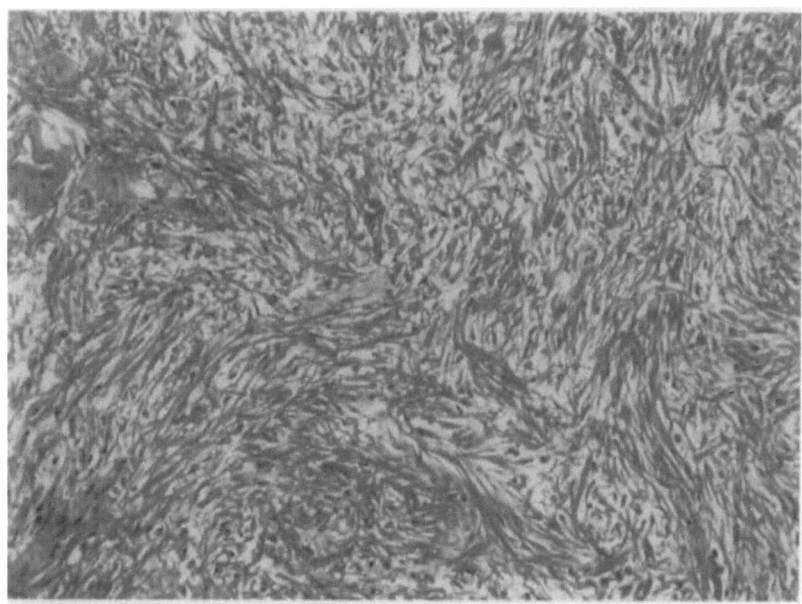

Fig. 105. *Astrocytoma*, optic nerve. Pilocytic glial cell and multiple Rosenthal fibres

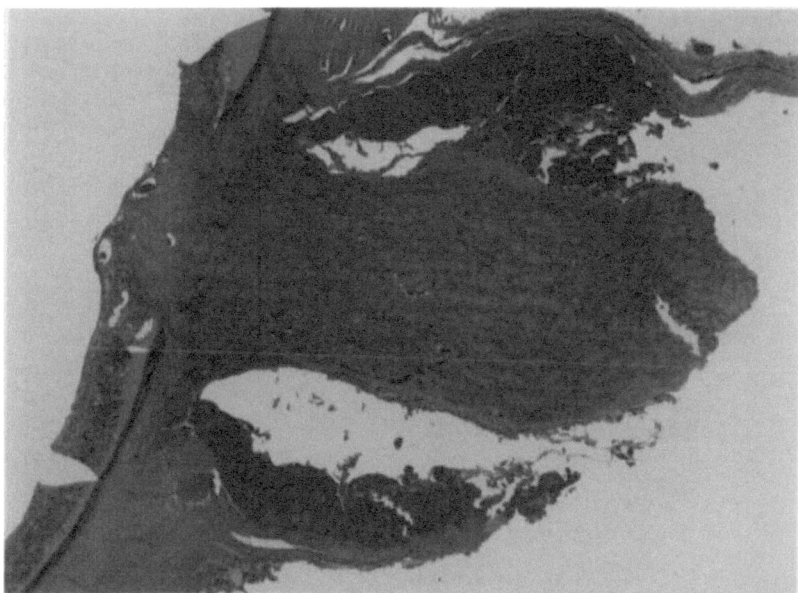

Fig. 106. *Meningioma,* optic nerve. Primary meningioma arises from arachnoid cells of optic nerve sheath

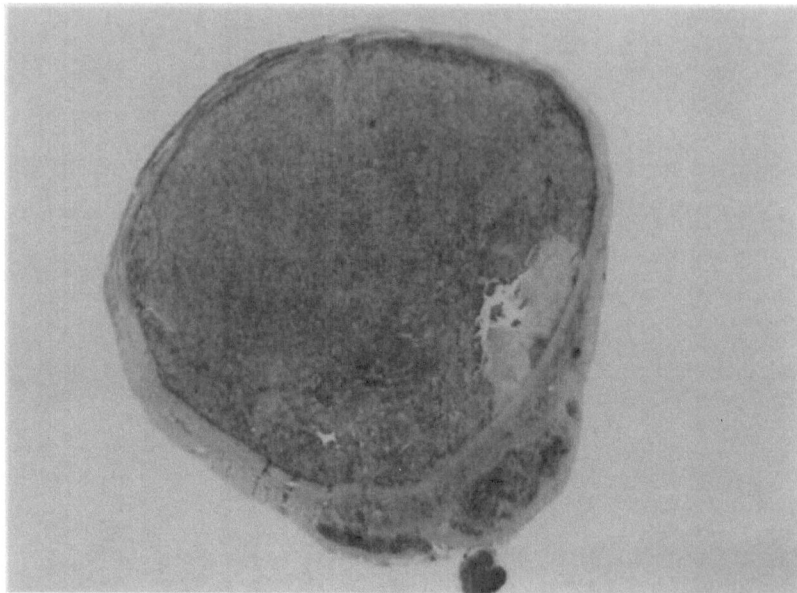

Fig. 107. *Meningioma*, optic nerve. Same tumour as in Fig. 106. Tumour cells surround optic nerve, causing compression

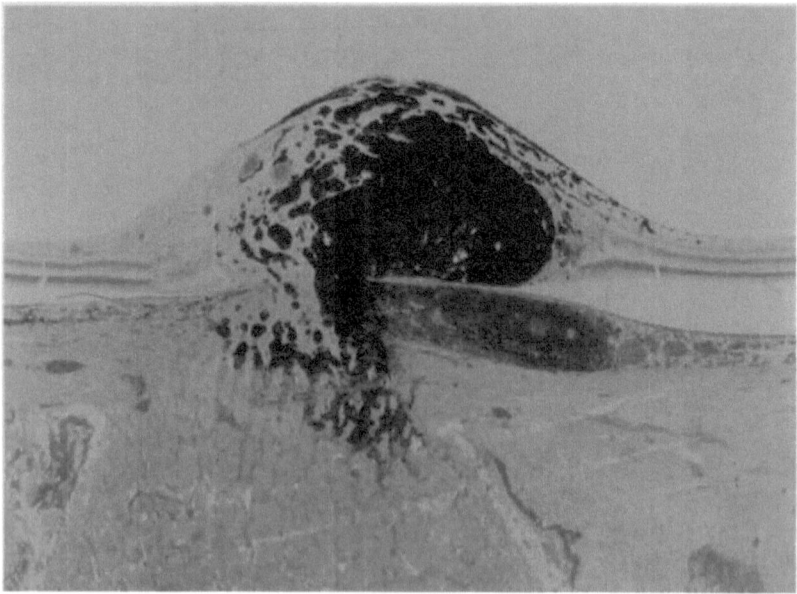

Fig. 108. *Melanocytoma*, optic disc. Darkly pigmented tumour cells extend into retina and optic nerve

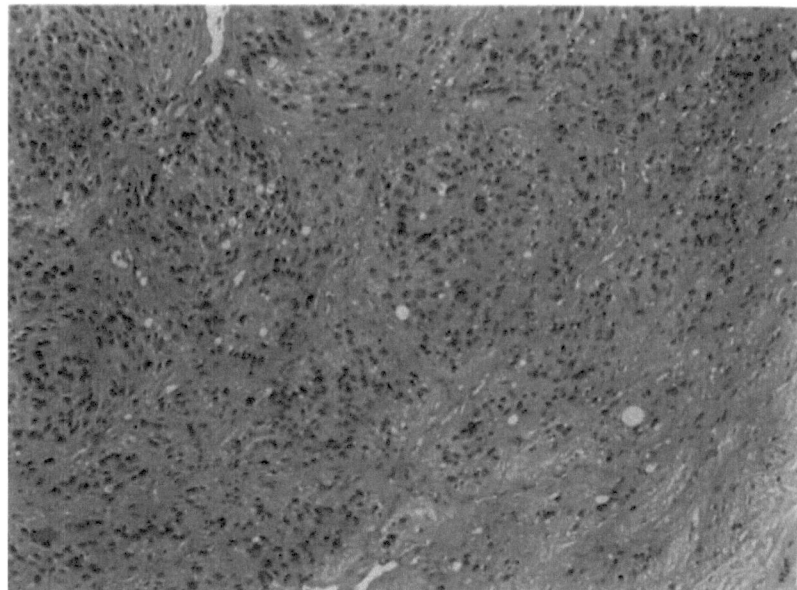

Fig. 109. *Gliobastoma multiforme,* optic nerve. Tumour has spread from a frontal lobe glioma

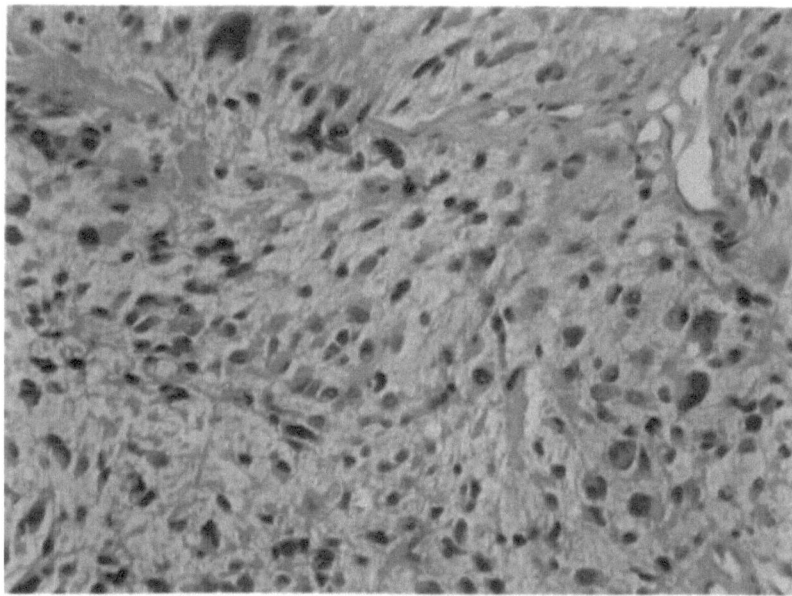

Fig. 110. *Glioblastoma multiforme,* optic nerve. Same tumour as in Fig. 109. Highly malignant large, anaplastic cells infiltrate nerve substance

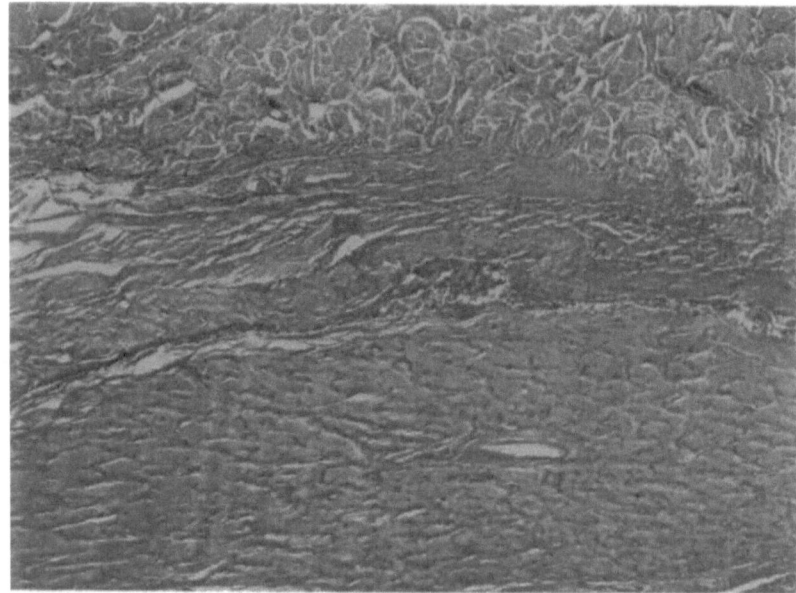

Fig. 111. *Meningioma*, orbit. A meningioma originating intracranially has extended into the orbit to surround the optic nerve

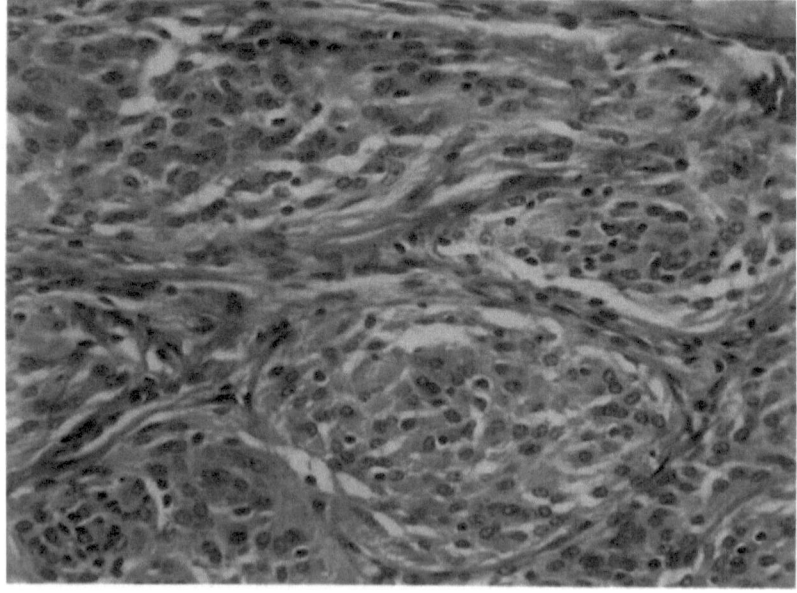

Fig. 112. *Meningioma*, optic nerve. Meningotheliomatous pattern consisting of rounded nests of proliferating arachnoid cells

Subject Index